W9-BEG-003

How to Prevent Your Stroke

How to Prevent
Your Stroke

J. David Spence, MD

Vanderbilt University Press

NASHVILLE

© 2006 Vanderbilt University Press
All rights reserved
First Edition 2006
10 09 08 07 06   2 3 4 5

Printed on acid-free paper.
Manufactured in the United States of America

Line drawings were prepared for this book by George Moogk,
a medical illustrator in London, Canada (Gem Graphics Inc.).
Text design by Dariel Mayer

The advice offered in this book, though based on the author's
experience with many thousands of patients, is not intended to be
a substitute for the advice and counsel of your personal physician,
and treatment should not be based solely on its contents.

Library of Congress Cataloging-in-Publication Data

Spence, J. David.
How to prevent your stroke / J. David Spence.
p. cm.
Includes bibliographical references and index.
ISBN-13: 978-0-8265-1536-0 (cloth : alk. paper)
ISBN-13: 978-0-8265-1537-7 (pbk. : alk. paper)
1. Cerebrovascular disease—Prevention. I. Title.
RC388.5.S66 2006
616.8'1—dc22
2005035450

Contents

Preface

Thirty years in a busy stroke-prevention clinic have convinced me that about 75 percent of strokes can be prevented in high-risk patients, and that many strokes occur needlessly because patients and doctors do not apply what we already know about preventing them.

The Revolution in Stroke Prevention

Whether you have already had a small warning stroke (a transient ischemic attack, or TIA), or whether you are at risk of stroke because of factors such as age, high blood pressure, artery disease, or family history, I hope you will read this book, find out what you need to know to prevent strokes, and put that knowledge into action.

A revolution in the treatment of acute stroke is under way right now, but the revolution in stroke prevention has already happened. We now know that lifestyle changes (particularly quitting smoking and adopting a healthy diet), detection and treatment of high blood pressure and high cholesterol, and, in some cases, surgery, markedly reduce the risk. We already have the weapons—effective, safe drugs and surgery for the right patients—but the war is going badly: every year, hundreds of thousands of people suffer the devastation of stroke unnecessarily because what we know is not being well enough applied.

I have yet to meet a person over age seventy who did not agree that death would be preferable to a bad stroke. More than death itself, most people fear a stroke's possible results: incapacity, incontinence, loss of speech, loss of independence, and burdening loved ones. However, in most cases the symptoms are transient, or the stroke is mild enough that a good recovery is likely. Treatment with the clot-buster drug tPA within three hours after the stroke—and the sooner the better—increases by 40 percent the chance of someone who has suffered a stroke going home without a severe disability.

Even better is the news that with the major advances in diagnosis and treatment developed in the past twenty years, about 75 percent of strokes can be prevented. In difficult cases, new approaches can make a big difference in controlling blood pressure, lowering cholesterol, and preventing arterial disease; all these approaches are described later in this book:

- The key to controlling difficult high blood pressure is a simple blood test to measure the activity in our body of one enzyme and one hormone: a kidney enzyme called renin, and an adrenal gland hormone called aldosterone.
- The levels of fat in the blood after a meal turn out to be more important than the level of cholesterol measured in a fasting cholesterol test, so we have, until recently, vastly underestimated the importance of a person's diet.
- Most people who have muscle problems from cholesterol-lowering drugs in the family called "statins" can resolve them by reducing the dose, adding ezetimibe (a generic drug marketed as Zetia or Ezetrol), and taking CoQ10, a dietary supplement.
- The most neglected treatable cause of artery disease is high levels of an amino acid called homocysteine, which can be treated with vitamins.

In rough order of importance, the measures we can take to prevent stroke are:

- Quitting smoking
- Controlling blood pressure
- Adhering to a Mediterranean diet (plus exercise)
- Taking cholesterol-lowering drugs

- Opening up blocked arteries
- Taking drugs that reduce blood clotting
- Treating homocysteine with vitamins

A person at high risk for stroke can reduce that risk by about 75 percent by putting all these preventive measures into action. Note that your doctor can help, but the biggest part of this is up to you. This becomes clearer when considering the time frame in which these measures reduce stroke.

A Quick Look at Preventive Measures

For smokers, quitting reduces the risk of stroke by about half within 6 months. Smoking is perhaps the most important risk factor for stroke because it is the only one that is entirely curable.

Effective control of blood pressure also reduces stroke risk by about half, but over several years. In difficult cases, getting control requires knowing the cause of the high blood pressure, in order to select the right treatment. This can easily be sorted out in most cases by measuring the blood levels of a kidney enzyme called renin, and an adrenal gland hormone called aldosterone. This approach is probably most important for people with African ancestry, who are much more likely to exhibit abnormal levels of these substances; without such tests, this cause of high blood pressure can easily be overlooked.

Regarding diet, a regimen that reduces stroke and heart attacks by about half within four years builds on the diet from the Mediterranean island of Crete. It is good for the arteries because it is high in beneficial substances such as olive oil, canola oil, the antioxidants in fruits and vegetables, and the fiber in whole grains, nuts, lentils and beans, and it is low in harmful substances such as cholesterol, trans fats, and animal fat. The trick to making it work is making it enjoyable. The appendix, which provides tips and recipes, is about learning how to do this.

Drugs that lower the level of cholesterol in the blood probably reduce by about 30 percent in four years the risk of any stroke, and by about 50 percent the risk of strokes due to atherosclerosis—plaque deposits, often called "hardening of the arteries"—as opposed to strokes due to high blood pressure. A diet low in salt and animal fat and high in fruits, vegetables, and low-fat dairy products also reduces blood pressure.

In certain cases, opening up blocked arteries via either surgery on the carotid (neck) artery or stenting (inserting a metal expanding sleeve into a narrowed artery to hold it open) reduces stroke risk substantially: in persons in whom the carotid artery is narrowed by 70 percent or more and who have had warning symptoms of stroke, surgically removing the inner layer of the artery with the plaque that is blocking the artery (endarterectomy)—reduces stroke or death by two-thirds over two years. (For patients with a narrow carotid artery who have not yet had warning symptoms of a stroke, I recommend surgery only for those at high risk of stroke, as evidenced by the particles breaking off the plaque (microemboli) that can be detected by ultrasound of the brain arteries (transcranial Doppler).

Drugs called anticoagulants, such as warfarin (a generic drug marketed as Coumadin and by other names), which reduce the production of clotting proteins, will reduce stroke risk by about half over one year in patients with atrial fibrillation (rapid, irregular heart contractions), and in other cases where clots are forming in the heart or veins and embolizing to the brain.

Other drugs that reduce clotting by interfering with blood platelets—so-called antiplatelet agents such as ASA (acetylsalicylic acid, or aspirin), clopidogrel (marketed as Plavix), or combination ASA/dipyridamole (marketed as Aggrenox)—will reduce stroke risk by about 25–30 percent in three to four years, but these will prevent only strokes due to embolization of platelet aggregates. They are not a panacea; stroke prevention requires figuring out what caused the small stroke, and then dealing with the cause. Doubling the dose of aspirin and crossing your fingers is not a useful approach to managing these.

Although I am not aware of evidence that exercise prevents stroke, it certainly reduces the risk of heart attacks, helps raise the level of HDL (the so-called good cholesterol), and improves diabetes and insulin resistance, so it is very likely that it will prevent stroke. About a half hour a day of brisk walking, or the equivalent, will get you most of the benefit of exercise.

The benefit of vitamin therapy for high levels of homocysteine is not yet proven; I hope the question will be resolved in the near future. A key issue for now is to treat vitamin B_{12} deficiency, which is much more common than most doctors believe.

If we add up the effects of all these interventions, we would reduce the risk of stroke by more than 100 percent, and obviously that doesn't work—there is some overlap among preventive measures. But I think a 75 percent reduction of stroke is a realistic goal, and that estimate coincides with an estimate published by my friend Phil Gorelick of Chicago, a stroke neurologist and U.S. leader in stroke prevention.

How This Book Is Organized

This book is divided into two main sections—what your doctor can do for you, and what you can do for yourself. I have also included a glossary of medical terms, an index of drug names (generic and trade names), and a section on healthful eating that contains gourmet recipes and tips for preparing enjoyable dishes.

A 75 percent reduction in your risk of stroke would be a wonderful outcome. I hope you adopt the recommendations you find in this book, and push yourself and your doctor to implement them.

Glossary of Medical Terms

aldosterone: a hormone from the outer part of the adrenal glands (which sit above each kidney, looking a bit like Napoleon's hat) that causes the kidney to retain salt and water, and excrete potassium. It also has other important effects relating to high blood pressure and artery disease.

amino acids: the building blocks that are strung together to make proteins. The sequence of amino acids in each protein is dictated by a gene. Our body can make most amino acids, but twelve must come from our diet, and so are called "essential amino acids."

angioplasty: the opening up of a narrowed artery by inflating a tiny balloon on the end of a thin plastic tube (a catheter) that has been inserted into an artery (often in the leg) and threaded up through the arterial system to the site of the blockage

angiotensin: a short chain of amino acids that constricts arteries, acts as a growth factor in the arteries and heart, and goes to the adrenal gland to cause it to release aldosterone

atherosclerosis: The underlying cause of heart attacks and most strokes, this condition is similar to the formation of scar tissue in the inner lining of the artery in response to injury. A focal buildup of atherosclerosis is called a plaque. It is much more than a deposit of fat and cholesterol in the artery wall.

atrium: either of the two upper chambers of the heart that receive blood from the veins and pump it into the ventricles

basilar artery: the main artery to the back part of the brain, formed by the two vertebral arteries joining up. It supplies blood to the brainstem and cerebellum, and then divides into

the two posterior cerebral arteries, which supply the back part
of the brain hemispheres – the occipital lobes and the inferior
mesial (interior) parts of the temporal lobes.

carotid arteries: the two main arteries at the front of the neck,
which supply blood to most of the brain (the cerebral
hemispheres)

circle of Willis: the natural bypass formed by a ring of arteries
at the base of the brain, connecting the carotid arteries to the
two posterior cerebral arteries. Named after Sir Thomas Willis,
who first described it about four hundred years ago.

embolus (plural, **emboli**): usually a chunk of artery wall, or a piece
of blood clot, that breaks off the artery wall or from the inner
lining of the heart and travels up through an artery into the
brain, lodging in a branch when it gets to one too small for it
to advance farther. Strokes due to emboli are called **embolic
strokes.**

endarterectomy: an operation to clean out a blocked artery;
usually a carotid artery

endothelium: the inner lining of the artery, an active organ that
produces substances that are both good for the artery (such as
nitric oxide) and bad for the artery (such as endothelin)

enzyme: a *protein* that speeds up chemical reactions in the body

fibrillation: very rapid, irregular, uncoordinated contractions of
the muscle fibers of the heart, resulting in loss of pumping
action of the part of the heart that is affected. In the case of
atrial fibrillation, this loss of pumping action allows blood to
pool in a side chamber of the left atrium called the auricle,
forming clots that can break off and cause strokes.

free radicals: chemically active compounds such as hydrogen
peroxide, with a free electron in the outer ring. These
substances can damage membranes, oxidize LDL cholesterol,
and do other harm to the arteries and the tissues supplied
by the arteries; they are often consumed in high-fat meals or
formed in chemical reactions with homocysteine and other
natural chemicals in the body.

homocysteine: an amino acid formed from methionine (found
mainly in meat), which increases clotting of the blood,
increases formation of free radicals, oxidizes cholesterol, and

damages the endothelium (the inner lining of the artery). High levels of homocysteine are associated with a high risk of stroke and heart attacks.

hormone: a regulatory chemical substance formed in one part of the body and carried by the blood to another part, where it affects cell activity

hypertension: high blood pressure

hypoglycemia: low blood sugar

hypokalemia: low level of potassium in the blood

incontinence: loss of control of bladder or bowel

infarction: permanent loss of blood flow that causes death of tissue, the result of obstruction of an artery by an embolus arriving at the site via the bloodstream, or a plaque rupture and consequent local clotting that blocks an artery

ischemia: sudden loss of blood flow to part of the brain because an artery supplying blood to that part of the brain has become blocked; may be temporary or permanent

ischemic stroke: a stroke (infarction) due to loss of blood supply to part of the brain

lipid: a fat or oil

magnetic resonance imaging (MRI): a technique that uses a powerful electromagnetic field that rapidly turns on and off, lining up atoms in the body and then allowing them to spin back. The spinning gives off waves like radio waves that can be detected and located by a powerful computer to make images of the brain and other organs.

magnetic resonance angiography (MRA): the injection of a contrast material (like a dye) that makes the arteries show up better on MRI; the computer can subtract the tissues around the arteries so they can be better visualized.

platelets: small cells that are packages of clotting activators, and travel in the bloodstream

statin: any of a class of drugs that reduce blood cholesterol levels by inhibiting a key enzyme (HMG Co A Reductase) involved in the formation of cholesterol, mainly in the liver. Blocking that enzyme also has other effects, including blocking with the formation of CoQ10 in the muscles.

stenosis: narrowing; usually refers to arteries, but may also refer to narrowing of other structures in the body

stenting: the insertion of a metal expanding sleeve into a narrowed artery to hold it open (and in the case of carotid stenting, to prevent chunks from breaking off and going up into the brain)

stroke: sudden loss of function of part of the brain

thrombus: a blood clot

TIA: transient ischemic attack; a small warning stroke

tPA: tissue plasminogen activator, a naturally occurring substance the body makes to dissolve clots. This can be manufactured and used as a clot-busting drug to open up blocked arteries in people who are experiencing a stroke or heart attack, but to be effective it has to be used soon after the artery becomes blocked.

transcranial Doppler (TCD): ultrasound beamed through the skull to assess flow in the arteries inside the head and to detect emboli (chunks) breaking off the carotid artery or other proximal sources of emboli

trans fat: harmful fats formed in prolonged heating of oils at high temperatures, or in the process of hydrogenating oils to make them solid. These are probably the most harmful of all fats, and should be avoided as much as possible by staying away from foods containing hydrogenated vegetable oils such as hard margarine, many commercial baked goods, and deep-fried foods.

vertebral arteries: the two arteries that run up through the bones at the back of the neck and supply the upper part of the spinal cord with blood; they then join to form the basilar artery.

vertebrobasilar ischemia: loss of blood supply to the part of the brain supplied by the vertebral and basilar arteries, and their branches, the posterior cerebral arteries.

Generic and Trade Drug Names

Drug Family / Class	Generic/Proper Name	Trade Name
Antihypertensive (to reduce blood pressure)		
ACE inhibitor	captopril	Capoten
	cilazapril	Inhibace
	enalapril	Vasotec
	fosinopril	Monopril
	lisinopril	Zestril
	quinapril	Accupril
	ramipril	Altace
	trandolapril	Mavik
ACE inhibitor plus diuretic	enalapril/HCTZ	Vasoretic
	lisinopril/HCTZ	Zestoretic
	perindopril/indapamide	Coversyl Plus
	quinapril/HCTZ	Accuretic
Beta blocker	acebutolol	Monitan
	atenolol	Tenormin
	metoprolol	Lopressor
	nadolol	Corgard
	pindolol	Visken
	propranolol	Inderal
	timolol	Blocadren
Beta blocker plus diuretic	atenolol-chlorthalidone	Tenoretic
	pindolol/HCTZ	Viskazide
Angiotensin receptor blocker (ARB)		
	candesartan	Atacand
	eposartan	Teveten
	irbesartan	Avapro
	losartan	Cozaar

Drug Family / Class	Generic/Proper Name	Trade Name
	telmisartan	Micardis
	valsartan	Diovan
ARB plus diuretic		
	candesartan/HCTZ	Atacand Plus
	eposartan/HCTZ	Teveten Plus
	irbesartan/HCTZ	Avalide
	telmisartan/HCTZ	Micardis Plus
	valsartan/HCTZ	Diovan Plus
Diuretic (to reduce water retention)		
	amiloride	Midamor
	chlorothalidone	Hygroton
	furosemide	Lasix
	hydrochlorothiazide (HCTZ)	Hydrodiuril, etc.
	indapamide	Lozide
	spironolactone	Aldactone
Diuretic combination	amiloride/HCTZ	Moduret
	atenolol/chlorothalidone	Tenoretic
	ethacrynic acid	Edecrine
	spironolactone/HCTZ	Aldactazide
	triamterene/HCTZ	Dyazide
Calcium channel blocker (to reduce blood pressure, heart pain, and arrhythmias)		
	amlodipine	Norvasc
	felodipine	Plendil
	nifedipine	Adalat
	nicardipine	Cardene
	verapamil	Isoptin, Chronovera
Alpha blocker (to block adrenaline receptors that constrict the arteries, called alpha receptors)		
	doxazosin	Cardura
	prazosin	Minipress
	terazosin	Hytrin
Peripheral vasodilator (to dilate the arteries)		
	hydralazine	Apresoline

Drug Family / Class	Generic/Proper Name	Trade Name

Antiplatelet agents (to block the clotting effects of blood platelets, which are like small packages of clotting agents traveling in the blood)

Drug Family / Class	Generic/Proper Name	Trade Name
Cyclo-oxygenase inhibitor	acetylsalicylic acid(ASA), aspirin	Aspirin, many brands
Thienopyridines	clopidogrel	Plavix
	ticlopidine	Ticlid
Phosphodiesterase inhibitor	dipyridamole	Persantine
Combination	dipyridamole/ASA	Aggrenox
Anticoagulant	heparin	Heparin
	warfarin	Coumadin
Low-molecular-weight heparin	enoxaparin	Lovenox
	dalteparin	Fragmin
	nadroparin	Fraxiparine
	tinzaparin	Innohep
	danaparoid	Organ
	fondaparinux	Arixtra

Cholesterol lowering

Drug Family / Class	Generic/Proper Name	Trade Name
Statins	atorvastatin	Lipitor
	fluvastatin	Lescol
	lovastatin	Mevacor
	pravastatin	Pravachol
	rosuvastatin	Crestor
	simvastatin	Zocor
Fibrates	bezafibrate	Bezalip
	fenofibrate	Lipidil
	gemfibrozil	Lopid
Niacin, slow-release	Niacin SR	Niaspan
Cholesterol absorption inhibitor	ezetimibe	Ezetrol, Ezetia

Bile-acid sequestrant

Drug Family / Class	Generic/Proper Name	Trade Name
	cholestyramine	Questran
	colestipol	Colestid
	psyllium mucilloid	Metamucil

Part 1
What Your Doctor Can Do

1
What Is a Stroke?

The Impending Epidemic

With the aging of the population, there is an impending epidemic of stroke, because stroke is so highly related to age. As Figure 1.1 shows, in the United States, strokes increase in a given year from 35 per 100,000 people at age thirty-five to 1,100 per 100,000 at ages seventy-five to eighty. If you are a baby boomer or older, you are arriving at the steep upslope of stroke risk, and you need to pay attention.

A stroke is the sudden loss of function of part of the brain. Usually, the cause is either (1) sudden loss of blood flow to part of the brain because an artery that supplies blood to that part of the brain has become blocked (ischemia), or (2) bleeding (hemorrhage) into the brain because an artery has burst.

In about 15 percent of individuals who come to an emergency room with the sudden onset of a brain disorder, the cause of stroke turns out to be an epileptic seizure followed by weakness on one side, or something else such as a brain tumor, low blood sugar (hypoglycemia), an abscess in the brain, a blood clot over the surface of the brain caused by head trauma, or some other condition.

Let's first look at how strokes happen when they are due to vascular, or blood-vessel, disease.

One of two kinds of vascular events causes strokes: a blocked artery, or a hemorrhage.

Strokes Due to Blocked Arteries

The brain is the organ that requires the most blood supply to function; when an artery to the brain is blocked, the territory supplied by that artery loses its oxygen, along with the fuel such as sugar that is

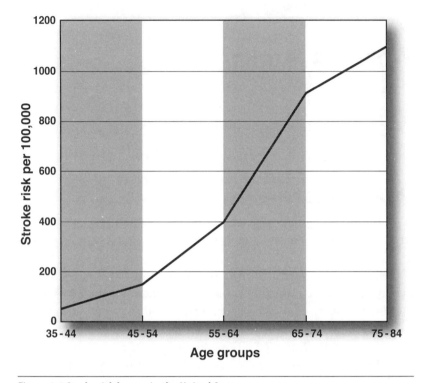

Figure 1.1 Stroke risk by age in the United States

required for brain function. This condition of deprivation of blood flow is called *ischemia*, so strokes due to blocked arteries are called *ischemic strokes*. If the blockage of the artery is long lasting, the part of the brain supplied by that artery is permanently damaged and dies; the damaged area is said to be *infarcted*, so ischemic strokes are also called *brain infarctions*, or *cerebral infarctions*. (Similarly, in heart attacks the heart muscle, the myocardium, is infarcted, so heart attacks are called *myocardial infarctions*.)

It is amazing how quickly the brain stops working when it loses its blood supply. When I was doing my rotation as a senior resident on the cardiology service, I had an opportunity to assess how long the brain can function without blood flow when we changed patients' pacemaker batteries: sometimes the heart stopped working until the new battery was plugged in. As I unplugged the old battery, I would ask the patient to start counting: nobody ever got past seven seconds.

If the blockage of the artery is temporary and blood flow is quickly restored, the brain recovers quickly. Most small warning strokes, called *transient ischemic attacks* or TIAs, last less than ten minutes. What happens is that an artery branch in the brain (like the branch of a tree) is temporarily blocked in one of three ways: by a clump of platelets (clotting activators that travel in the bloodstream), a chunk of artery wall, or a clump of blood clot.

The chunk comes through the bloodstream, either from the large artery in the neck (like the trunk of the tree) or from the heart. These chunks that have arisen in the heart or large arteries and that travel through the bloodstream until they lodge in branches that are too small for them to pass are called *emboli*. Thus, strokes due to emboli are called *embolic strokes*. This term is usually used to describe strokes caused by large blood clots from the heart, but in fact, when blood pressure is controlled, emboli from the artery wall cause most strokes.

Clumps of Platelets

The first kind of blockage, emboli arising from the artery wall, is of two main types: either clumps of platelets or chunks of debris from plaques in the artery wall due to atherosclerosis—that is, blocked arteries (atherosclerotic debris).

Smaller than red blood cells, platelets are like small bags of clotting activators that travel in the bloodstream. When platelets are brushed or smashed against the artery wall by flow disturbances such as turbulence (like a kayak that hits a rock in the rapids), they release substances that cause the platelets to stick to the wall and form clumps. The clumps, which have a white doughy appearance, can then break off from the artery wall and travel in the bloodstream until they get lodged in a branch that is too small for them to pass through. If the clump oozes through or breaks up, blood flow is restored, and the symptoms are only temporary.

A blood clot is called a *thrombus*, and formation of a clot is called *thrombosis*: because platelet clumps are white, they are sometimes called *white thrombus*. Acetylsalicylic acid (ASA, or aspirin) and

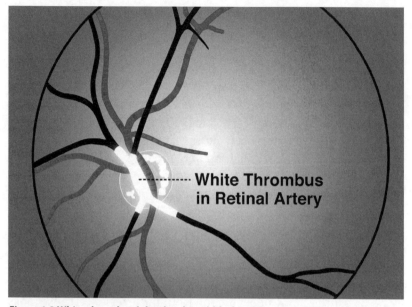

Figure 1.2 White thrombus (platelet clump) blocking the central artery of the retina (at the back of the eye)

newer drugs that prevent platelet clumping are called *antiplatelet agents*. (*Blood thinners* is a misnomer; these drugs don't thin the blood, they reduce formation of clots.)

I have twice been on the scene when an individual experienced sudden loss of vision due to blockage of the main artery to the eye by a platelet clump (Figure 1.2). Because the arteries at the back of the eye can be seen directly through a scope designed for looking in eyes (an ophthalmoscope), it was possible to watch what happened as the platelet clump oozed through the artery like dough, gradually working its way into the branches in smaller pieces and then disappearing; when the embolus was gone, vision returned within seconds.

Plaque Chunks

If the material that blocks the artery in the eye or brain is of the second type, a chunk of atherosclerotic plaque, it may work its way through the artery to a small branch, with recovery of function as the blood flow is restored via other small artery branches—or the branch that is blocked may be large enough that loss of blood flow to the part of the brain it supplies may be permanent. When this happens in the eye, an observer with an ophthalmoscope can see, for some days to weeks after the event, a bright spot in the retina of the eye; its shininess comes from cholesterol crystals in the chunk of plaque reflecting the light from the instrument. (This is called a *Hollenhorst plaque*, named after the first person to describe it.)

Blood-Clot Chunks

The third main type of embolus is a chunk of blood clot that forms in the heart. Blood clots that form in slow-moving blood, or in settings where blood flow is stagnant, are quite different from platelet clumps. This kind of clot is called *red thrombus*. It involves a different process, which is important because the treatment is different. Red thrombus forms when strands of fibrin, a blood-clotting protein, grow longer and longer, forming a mesh like fiberglass wool. The mesh entraps red blood cells and platelets and tends to keep growing. The red blood cells give the clot a red appearance.

The drugs used to prevent red thrombus act by reducing the levels of blood-clotting proteins, thus preventing the coagulation of the blood, so they are called *anticoagulants*. The two main types are heparin, which is given by injection, and warfarin (Coumadin), which is taken in pill form. (Under development are new anticoagulant pills, which do not require frequent blood tests to adjust the dose but do require occasional blood testing because the early ones under development can affect the liver in about 7 percent of people; monitoring is required to detect this problem so the drug can be stopped before liver damage occurs. Undoubtedly there will be new safer variants developed in future.)

Strokes Due to Hemorrhage

Strokes due to bleeding into the brain (intracerebral hemorrhage) or into the space between the brain and the inner lining of the skull (subarachnoid hemorrhage) account for about 20 percent of stroke in locales where blood pressure is well controlled, and up to 40 percent where it is not.

High Blood Pressure

The commonest type of brain hemorrhage is due to high blood pressure. These hemorrhages go into the deep part of the brain, near the base, and are caused by rupture of small artery branches, or *arterioles*. They happen because high blood pressure damages the arterioles in two ways (lipohyaline degeneration and fibrinoid necrosis); this damage is distinct from atherosclerosis (the main cause of heart attacks or strokes due to large artery disease, as we see in Chapter 3). These hemorrhages can be almost completely prevented by good control of blood pressure.

In the North American Symptomatic Carotid Endarterectomy (NASCET) trial (described in more detail later), we tried very hard to control blood pressure, and reduced hemorrhagic stroke to less than 1 percent of stroke—a great improvement over the average of about 30 percent in most locales at the time (1). Controlling blood pressure also prevents strokes due to blockage of small arterioles, called lacunar infarctions because they look under the microscope like tiny lagoons. For the most part, then, preventing brain hemorrhage is about effective blood-pressure control, and preventing lacunar strokes is also mainly about blood pressure control, so a large part of this book is devoted to effective strategies toward that end: diagnosing the underlying cause of high blood pressure so that the right medications can be used to control blood pressure and reduce their adverse effects.

Surgery—Or Not

Another method to prevent hemorrhage, besides controlling high blood pressure, is surgery for blood-vessel abnormalities that can cause hemorrhage when the arteries or veins rupture.

AVMS

In arteriovenous malformations (AVMs), arteries flow directly into veins instead of going through tiny branches called capillaries, so the pressure in the veins is higher than in normal veins, and they may rupture. AVMs may require surgery, or sometimes they can be treated by putting a narrow tube (a catheter) up into the brain arteries from an artery in the leg, and injecting a form of superglue or releasing little balloons to block the arteries leading to the AVM.

ANEURYSMS

Aneurysms (areas of artery that bulge due to a weakness in the wall of the artery, like a bulge in the wall of a tire) often look like small red berries, so they are called *berry aneurysms*. They tend to be located at places where arteries branch at the base of the brain, around the circle of Willis (see Figure 2.1). When they rupture, they cause an abrupt severe headache, like an explosion, sometimes called a *thunderclap headache*. Often a person grabs his or her head and cries out; it is typically described as "the worst headache I ever had in my life."

Because the ruptured aneurysm can often be treated successfully to prevent a fatal rebleed, it is important that the condition be diagnosed. The diagnosis typically involves first a brain X-ray such as a CT scan, and if the CT scan is negative, a spinal tap to make sure there is no blood in the spinal fluid. Aneurysms can be treated surgically by putting a clip on the neck of the aneurysm, but many can be treated through a catheter, by putting a small balloon or platinum coils into the aneurysm so that it will clot and be rendered safe.

Berry aneurysms can be familial and are sometimes associated with a hereditary condition called *polycystic kidney disease,* which means multiple cysts have formed in the kidney. If there is a family history of the disease, it may be appropriate for family members to be screened with tests such as magnetic resonance angiography (MRA). The problem is what to do when unruptured aneurysms are discovered. Recent studies show that small aneurysms are very unlikely to rupture, and until aneurysms are bigger than about nine millimeters, the risk of rupture is lower than the risk associated with surgery (2). Because aneurysms may enlarge over time, repeat MRA tests may be required at intervals of about a year to monitor their size.

CAVERNOMAS

Another cause of small strokes due to hemorrhage is cavernous angiomas, called *cavernomas,* which consist mainly of thin-walled veins in a small cluster that on an MRI (magnetic resonance imaging) scan looks like popcorn. They seldom cause large hemorrhages because the pressure in the veins is low, but they often cause epileptic seizures because they may leak a small amount of blood, which is very irritating to the cortex (outer layer) of the brain. These lesions may be hereditary, are more common in Hispanic Americans (3), particularly of Mexican origin, and may be multiple. Only rarely may they be treated surgically, because when there are many lesions or they are in critical locations, surgery may be impractical. Radiation is a possible alternative, but often the appropriate course is no treatment.

Lobar Hemorrhages

Hemorrhages under the brain's outer layer, the cortex, called *lobar hemorrhages,* are often due in elderly individuals to a weakening of the arteries by deposits of a protein called amyloid. This condition is called *amyloid angiopathy* (*angiopathy* is the generic term for any disease of the *blood vessels*). The hemorrhages are not caused by high blood pressure, and at present there is no way to prevent them, but because amyloid is also involved in Alzheimer's disease, there is a lot of research under way, and it seems likely that effective therapy for this condition may appear before long.

2
Symptoms and Signs

Small Warning Strokes:
Transient Ischemic Attacks (TIAs)

Individuals and their physicians need to understand that just because symptoms last only a few minutes, it doesn't mean that the problem with the arteries is minor. In fact, a complete blockage of the carotid artery (the main artery that carries blood to the front part of the brain) can occur without any symptoms or can present just as a headache, or a brief episode of weakness or numbness on one side; nevertheless, that blockage may lead to a severe stroke that progresses to brain swelling and death in three or four days.

Brief episodes of loss of blood supply to part of the brain are called *transient ischemic attacks*, or TIAs; usually they last only minutes, but sometimes they last several hours. The reason for this variability is that there are backup sources of blood supply to the brain, all connected by a circle, much like a ring road or natural bypass underneath the brain, called the circle of Willis.

The problem is that if a minor episode occurs, individuals and their doctors tend to conclude it was caused by a minor problem. Even if they realize that the episode represented a TIA, there is a tendency to minimize it, and for your physician to suggest that you "take an aspirin and cross your fingers."

This is a huge mistake. In a way, a TIA or warning stroke, is the ultimate medical emergency. It represents a golden window of opportunity to prevent a more serious stroke and should be followed up with tests to find its cause. This is vital, because the appropriate treatment to prevent another (possibly major) stroke depends on

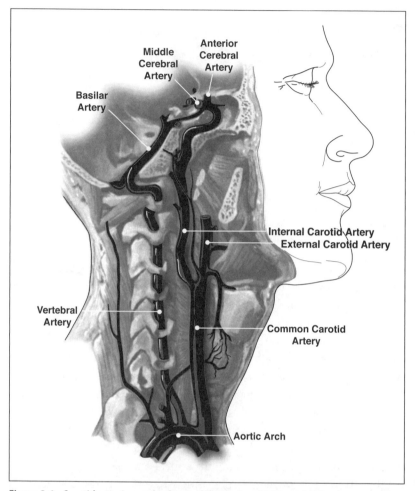

Figure 2.1a Carotid arteries at the front of the neck, which supply blood to most of the brain, and vertebral arteries at the back of the neck, which supply blood to the upper part of the spinal cord, then join to form the basilar artery

what that cause was. About 15 percent of people who look as if they have had a stroke have had something else, not related to arteries (discussed later). About 20 percent of cerebral infarctions (damage to brain tissue due to loss of blood supply) are due to blood clots breaking off from the heart and moving (embolizing) to the brain. Those cases need treatment with anticoagulants (anticlotting agents), not aspirin.

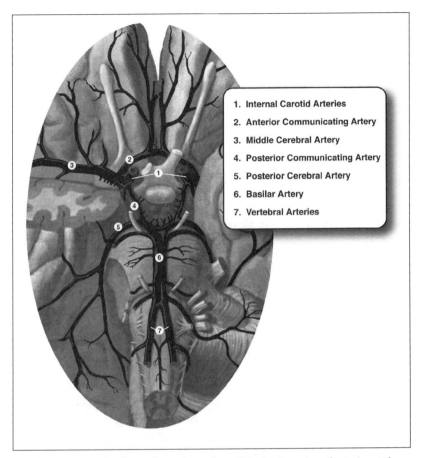

1. Internal Carotid Arteries
2. Anterior Communicating Artery
3. Middle Cerebral Artery
4. Posterior Communicating Artery
5. Posterior Cerebral Artery
6. Basilar Artery
7. Vertebral Arteries

Figure 2.1b Circle of Willis on the undersurface of the brain, a ring of arteries at the base of the brain connecting the carotid arteries to the two posterior cerebral arteries, providing backup blood supply to the brain

If the stroke or TIA was due to emboli of platelet clumps from the artery in the neck, antiplatelet agents such as acetylsalicylic acid (aspirin, ASA), are indicated. Adding additional antiplatelet agents (such as dipyridamole/ASA or clopidogrel) makes only a small difference. However, if the stroke or TIA was due to emboli of chunks of plaque from a severe narrowing of the carotid artery in the neck, then antiplatelet agents are less likely to work, and an operation to clean out the artery is indicated, as we discuss later.

It is important, therefore, to recognize small strokes or TIAs when they occur, since this recognition is what triggers the next step—finding out what caused it.

Diagnosing the cause of a TIA is like detective work: it involves trying to figure out what part of the brain was affected, and what caused the transient loss of blood supply to produce the symptoms that happened. To recognize that the symptoms were due to a transient blockage of a brain artery, they need to be localized to a part of the brain that is supplied by one of the major arteries to the brain.

First, though, it is important to rule out other possibilities: causes that mimic vascular stroke.

Other Problems That Might Be Confused with a Vascular Stroke

Among the people who arrive at an emergency room looking like they have a vascular stroke, about 15 percent actually have something else.

Hypoglycemia (Low Blood Sugar)

The very first individual I saw with a stroke was in the emergency room on my first day as an intern. My beeper went off as I was going into the hospital cafeteria to grab some supper. The doctor in the emergency room who had paged me could hear the noises in the background and said, "Don't rush your supper; it's just a stroke." I put down my tray and went over to the ER right away.

The patient was a seventy-year-old man from the nearby Oneida Indian reservation who came in unconscious, with paralysis of his right side. Because diabetes is very common in the First Nations people, the history, obtained from his wife, went like this: "Is he diabetic?" "Yes." "Has he taken his insulin today?" "Yes, I gave it to him at seven o'clock this morning." "How much insulin does he take?" "Seventy units." "Has he eaten today?" "No, we found him unconscious on the floor at five o'clock this afternoon, and his breakfast was still on the table."

I drew a blood sample to measure the sugar level and gave the man a dose of sugar injected into a vein. He sat up, asked for a drink of water, took it with his previously paralyzed right hand, drank some, and said "Christ, that's cold!" I introduced him to the ER doctor who had referred him, and began my lifelong passion for stroke prevention. His blood sugar came back very low, confirming that his "stroke" was due to low blood sugar (hypoglycemia). Since then I have seen only two other patients whose apparent stroke was due to hypoglycemia, so it's not common, but definitely an important consideration because, first, the treatment is so easy, and, second, overlooking this cause can be disastrous

Like this man, a small number of people who seem to have had strokes will have a reversible metabolic condition such as hypoglycemia. We don't yet understand clearly how a metabolic disturbance can produce signs localized to one part of the brain.

Seizure

Similar confusion can occur when a person complains after an epileptic seizure of weakness of part of the body, such as an arm, or of one side of the body. This is called *postictal paralysis*, (*-ictal* means "related to seizure") and is perhaps the commonest mimic of vascular stroke. The mechanism may relate to metabolic exhaustion of the part of the brain that was most involved in the seizure; neurons fire hundreds of times per second during epileptic events, and in addition to exceeding the capacity of the arterial blood flow to provide adequate nutrients and oxygen to sustain such a fury, they also build up acid and metabolic waste products that exceed the capacity of the venous system to carry them away.

Brain tumors can sometimes cause sudden weakness that suggests a stroke; such occurrences may be related to swelling after a minor head injury, a hemorrhage into the tumor, or a seizure related to the tumor, with postictal paralysis perhaps aggravated by swelling. Brain abscesses can mimic a stroke in much the same way that a tumor can, but these are more readily cured with surgical drainage and antibiotics.

Loss of Consciousness

Interruption of blood flow to the brain can cause loss of consciousness. This may be due to a problem with blood flow to the back of the brain (the vertebral/basilar arteries), so it can be a symptom of stroke (especially if associated with other symptoms pointing to the back of the brain), but more commonly it is due to interruption of blood flow to the whole brain. The word *blackout* is a diagnostic trap. It may mean either transient loss of vision or transient loss of consciousness. Often loss of vision precedes loss of consciousness; I suspect that's why we call loss of consciousness a blackout.

The commonest cause of loss of consciousness is a temporary drop in blood pressure, with interruption of the blood supply to the whole brain. This is called fainting, or *syncope* (pronounced "sin-co-pee"). This may be due to a heart rhythm disturbance, which could require a pacemaker or other intervention. The problem usually results from blood dropping into the major veins of the legs when one stands up quickly, with a drop in blood pressure. Because there is a change in posture involved, this kind of fainting is called *postural hypotension* (abnormally low blood pressure), or *postural syncope.*

Someone who faints typically first feels lightheaded, then as if everything is going far away, along with roaring in the ears, dimming and then loss of vision, and afterward waking up on the floor. Observers may see that the person is pale and sweaty.

In healthy young people, a shock such as the sight of blood may cause fainting, with a slowing of the heart and dilation of the blood vessels. The problem can be quite impressive; a needle inserted into a vein for blood sampling so shocked a patient of one of my colleagues, David Boyd, that the patient's heart stopped for twenty-six seconds.

Fainting as a result of shock sometimes is accompanied by a brief seizure. (This seems to happen more often when a woman faints upon insertion of an intrauterine device; half a dozen patients of my wife, a family doctor, have had this experience.)

Common reasons for postural hypotension include dehydration from excessive sweating or diarrhea, diabetic nerve damage (neuropathy), and medications that interfere with the reflexes controlling blood pressure, such as antidepressant drugs. Potassium depletion from diuretics, and some of the blood-pressure drugs that are no longer used much (such as guanethidine and methyldopa), also can cause this kind of fainting. A fairly common cause that is often missed is a recent heart attack, if it occurred without pain. (About 40 percent of heart attacks are "silent" because they are not associated with the typical crushing chest pain; the victim may faint, or feel weak and sweaty, or even vomit and have diarrhea, which can be mistaken for food poisoning, because of disturbance of autonomic control.)

Some specific situations that can lead to fainting are prolonged violent coughing (cough syncope), and a drop in blood pressure after emptying of the bladder (micturition syncope).

Blood Clots

A blood clot under the lining of the skull, a *subdural hematoma*, sometimes can produce symptoms that mimic vascular stroke. These blood clots usually result from a head injury that ruptures a vein running from the surface of the brain to the inner lining of the skull. After the initial hemorrhage, the clot occupies the space between the brain and the skull; it tends to enlarge because the remaining bridging veins are stretched and therefore more likely to rupture. A membrane grows around the clot, forming a kind of sac, and the clot grows because as the blood breaks down it draws water into the sac. As the clot enlarges, it may cause headaches and diffuse symptoms such as confusion and difficulty walking; when symptoms are localized to the part of the brain underlying the clot, this can mimic a stroke, especially if the individual is confused and cannot give a good history of the symptoms that preceded the development of focal signs.

Migraine

Migraine is especially tricky: it can mimic a stroke, and it can also be associated with strokes. It used to be thought that the warning symptoms or "aura" of migraine was due to spasm of the blood vessels in part of the brain; it now seems likely that a form of electrical dysfunction may be more important. Typically, the attack starts with flashing lights, zigzag lines, or a dark spot in one's field of vision, then go on to a severe throbbing headache, followed by vomiting. In some cases the aura may include numbness and weakness on one side of the body, or loss of speech, so that a stroke is suspected.

One thing that makes diagnosis tricky is that not all migraine attacks are associated with headache; another is that individuals with migraine are twice as likely to have a heart-valve condition called *mitral prolapse* that can cause small blood clots to form on the heart's mitral valve; these can break off and go to the brain, actually causing a small stroke. When this happens in a young person with migraine, it is often blamed on "migraine without headache," or on the birth-control pill and migraine, because women are twice as likely as men to have mitral prolapse. Individuals with migraine are also more likely to have a hole in the dividing wall between the two upper chambers of the heart (the atria). This predisposes them to a type of stroke called paradoxical embolism, discussed in a later chapter.

Vertigo or Dysequilibrium

People experiencing vertigo or dysequilibrium often say they feel "dizzy." But your doctor needs specifics. Do you feel faint or light-headed when you stand up (denoting a drop in blood pressure)? Do you feel as if you are spinning, or things around you are spinning (vertigo)? Do you feel as if you were on a rocking boat (dysequilibrium)? Do you stagger when you walk (ataxia)? And so on.

Each inner ear has a balance gizmo called the *vestibular apparatus*. It is an arrangement of three semicircular canals, each oriented in a different plane, so that movement of the body or head causes fluid in one of the canals to move and send a signal to the brain.

The commonest causes of vertigo or dysequilibrium are inner ear problems such as labyrinthitis (an acute inflammation of the balance mechanism of the inner ear, possibly related to viral infection) or cupulolithiasis (grains of debris like tiny stones in the fluid of the inner ear). The signal your brain gets from each inner ear has to be exactly reciprocal: if you turn your head to the left, the brain gets a signal from the right ear that it went forward so far, at a certain speed, for so long; the left ear simultaneously signals that it went backward. The signal from the left ear has to match the right one exactly. If the signal from one inner ear is either more or less intense than the signal from the other side, you feel a sensation of rotation or movement, often with nausea and staggering (ataxia). Sometimes a visual symptom that is caused by jerking of the eyes makes everything seem to be jerking from side to side, and it is difficult to focus. This symptom, called *oscillopsia*, corresponds to a physical sign called nystagmus (the eyes jerking rhythmically) that can be observed by others. These symptoms by themselves (vertigo, nausea, vomiting, ataxia, oscillopsia) are seldom due to a stroke; they are almost always due to an inner ear problem.

As we will see, vertigo or dysequilibrium may be symptoms of a stroke if they are associated with a constellation of other specific symptoms.

Stroke Syndromes

Symptoms that can be traced to the territory of a major artery to the brain, and that should lead to the diagnosis of TIA, include transient blindness in one eye, speech disturbance, weakness and/or numbness of one side of the body, loss of consciousness, vertigo (when it occurs with other symptoms), and various problems with vision and memory.

Transient Blindness in One Eye

The artery that supplies blood to the eye (ophthalmic artery) is a branch of the internal carotid artery (the main artery that carries blood to the front part of the brain). For that reason, symptoms in only one eye are a predictor of increased risk of strokes on that side of the brain (and the opposite side of the body).

A typical attack would involves sudden loss of vision in one eye, recovering over minutes. This is called *amaurosis fugax*, which translates as "fleeting blindness." Sometimes vision will be interrupted, or will recover, in only half the field of vision (the top or bottom, or the left or right side of the field). To the individual, it may seem as if a curtain falls or rises to block the vision, and then is lifted or pulled aside. Some people say the experience is like looking through water on one lens of their eyeglasses, or like the foggy or frosted appearance of the back of a mirror.

It is important to distinguish between loss of vision in one eye and loss of vision in one half of the visual field, because this is what determines where the problem is coming from.

What can confuse the diagnosis is that our visual pathways are crossed: we see the things that are off to our right with the left half of the brain, and vice-versa (see Figure 2.2). If the problem is in only one eye, it originated in the carotid artery on the same side; if the loss of vision is off to one side in both eyes, it may be from a problem in the vertebral arteries or the basilar artery, which together supply blood to the back part of the brain on the side of the brain opposite the visual loss. Getting the diagnosis wrong could lead to an unnecessary operation on a narrowed carotid artery that is not causing symptoms (i.e., it is asymptomatic). The issue of surgery for asymptomatic carotid narrowing, or stenosis, is discussed in a later chapter.

If you are not sure, it is better to be aware that there is uncertainty rather than to make assumptions. Similar confusion can occur with speech disturbances.

Speech Disturbance

Difficulty with speech can originate from either carotid artery, or from the vertebral/basilar arteries. Sorting out which side is involved is important, as the treatment for each may be different: if the problem is due to severe narrowing of the carotid artery on one side, an operation to clean out the artery is indicated. On the other hand, if it is due to blockage of the basilar artery, treatment with anticoagulants such as warfarin (Coumadin) may be indicated.

There are two main kinds of speech disturbance: a disorder of language, called *aphasia*, and a problem with pronouncing words clearly, called *dysarthria*. It can be quite tricky at times to sort this out; this problem is particularly difficult because the two sometimes occur together.

A common mistake is made by many doctors who think the issue can be sorted out by the question, "Did you know what you wanted to say but couldn't say it?" The diagnosis of aphasia depends instead on whether the individual made mistakes in grammar, or said wrong words, or could not understand what was being said. Difficulty in finding the names of objects may lead to saying wrong nouns, or "talking around the noun," which is also called *circumlocu-*

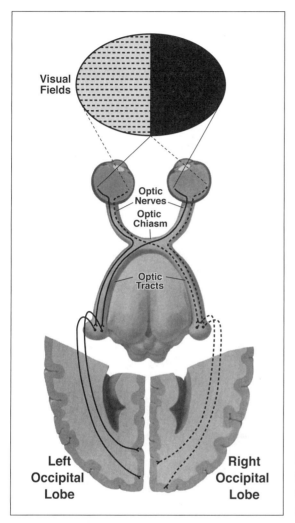

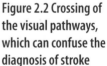

Figure 2.2 Crossing of the visual pathways, which can confuse the diagnosis of stroke

tion; for example, instead of correctly naming a pen, an individual with aphasia may call it a pencil or describe it as "something to write with." Some words may be combined or slightly garbled. If there are errors in comprehension or grammar, or wrong words are coming out, the problem is aphasia, which is usually due to a problem in the left side of the brain. (About 50 percent of left-handed people, who represent about 15 percent of the population—that is, 7.5 percent of all individuals—may have important language function on the right side of the brain, but the rest, which is almost everyone, have most of their language function on the left side.)

If the problem is strictly thickened speech, like that of a drunk, with no difficulty in understanding and no errors in grammar or words, then the problem is dysarthria (thickening of speech), which can come from either carotid artery or from the arteries at the back of the brain. In that circumstance, we try to determine what part of the brain is affected from associated symptoms such as numbness or weakness on one side.

Weakness and Numbness on One Side

Transient blockage of the carotid artery or of its major branches, the anterior and middle cerebral arteries, commonly causes weakness and numbness on the opposite side of the body (face, arm, and leg). This may be accompanied by thickening of speech from either side, or by aphasia, if it is the carotid artery on the dominant side (usually the left). Occasionally the numbness or weakness may spare the face or leg; rarely, if the anterior cerebral artery alone is affected, the leg alone may be affected. Ischemia (blocked blood flow) in the brainstem due to a problem with the vertebral arteries or basilar artery may cause numbness or weakness down one side of the body, but commonly the symptoms have a variation such as numbness on both sides of the face, or around the mouth, or the face on one side and the arm and leg on the opposite side.

When numbness or weakness affects only the leg, then the problem may be in the spinal cord or in the nerve roots in the lower back—the sciatic nerve or one of its branches—so it is not so easy to be sure it is a TIA. Similarly, numbness in one hand alone is commonly from a problem with the median nerve (carpal tunnel syndrome) or from a disc in the neck that affects a nerve root that goes down the arm or the nerve that winds around the elbow, the ulnar nerve (often referred to as the "funny bone" because it causes an electrical sensation down your arm if you bang your elbow on something).

Weakness in both legs simultaneously, particularly if accompanied by trouble with bladder control, often indicates a problem in the spinal cord; this is also an important emergency. (When the spinal cord is causing symptoms, it is like a flickering candle: if it goes out, it usually cannot be relit. When something is compressing the spinal cord and causing symptoms, the compression must be relieved soon to avoid permanent paralysis.)

Sensory and Visual "Neglect"

An interesting problem that happens more with strokes on the right side of the brain is called "neglect." The person may not be aware of weakness or loss of vision off to one side, or of loss of sensation on one side. This lack of awareness can be so extreme that if the paralyzed hand is held up in front of the face, the person may deny ownership of the hand. This phenomenon is partly responsible for delayed diagnosis of strokes in the right hemisphere: if the person is not aware that there is a problem, it will not be reported to family or bystanders. It is important to approach people with this problem from the side of the world they can see.

Loss of Consciousness, Vertigo, or Dysequilibrium

Vertigo or dysequilibrium may be symptoms of a stroke if they are associated with other symptoms such as numbness, tingling, weakness, thickening of speech (dysarthria), double vision (diplopia), flashing lights in the vision, loss of vision, or problems with memory.

Constellations of Symptoms

In individuals who have a TIA, or small warning stroke, a specific constellation of symptoms points to reduced blood flow in the network of arteries that serve the back of the brain. The arteries that run up through the bones in the back of the neck are the vertebral arteries. The vertebral arteries penetrate the base of the skull, and then join up to form the basilar artery (see Figure 2.1a), which supplies the brainstem. Then the basilar artery branches to form the two posterior cerebral arteries, which supply the back part of the brain (the occipital lobes), and the inferior mesial (underneath, toward the center) temporal lobes (see Figure 2.1b). The blood vessels supplying this part of the brain are called called the *vertebrobasilar system*.

The particular constellation of symptoms an individual experiences points to which part of the brain and which arteries are involved in the reduction of blood flow (see Figure 2.3).

Visual symptoms (flashing lights, zigzag lines, loss of vision in both eyes or in the visual field off to one side) point to involvement of the occipital lobes. Impaired visual processing—for example, being unable to recognize familiar faces, or becoming lost in familiar surroundings—indicates involvement of the nearby cortex that serves visual association. Permanent impairment of short-term memory suggests permanent damage in both temporal lobes; temporary impairment of short-term memory, which is called *transient global amnesia*, points to temporary loss of blood flow to the mesial temporal lobes. During an episode of transient global amnesia an individual may be alert and seem to function normally but cannot record ongoing memory; typically the person asks the same question over and over again (e.g., "Why are we here?" or "What are we doing?") and later has no recollection of the episode, which may go on for hours.

Double vision points to involvement of the top part of the brainstem (the midbrain); vertigo or facial numbness, to involvement in the middle part (the pons); and thickening of speech (dysarthria) and trouble with swallowing to the lowest part (the medulla). Numbness and weakness on one side or both sides of the body may occur when lesions in any part of the brainstem affect the nerves that run from the spinal cord to the brain, or vice-versa. Clumsiness and staggering suggest involvement of the cerebellum.

Sudden loss of blood flow to the cranial nerve nuclei and their connections in the brainstem may cause facial numbness and weakness, double vision, difficulty swallowing, thickness of speech, vertigo, tinnitus (ringing in the ears), and deafness.

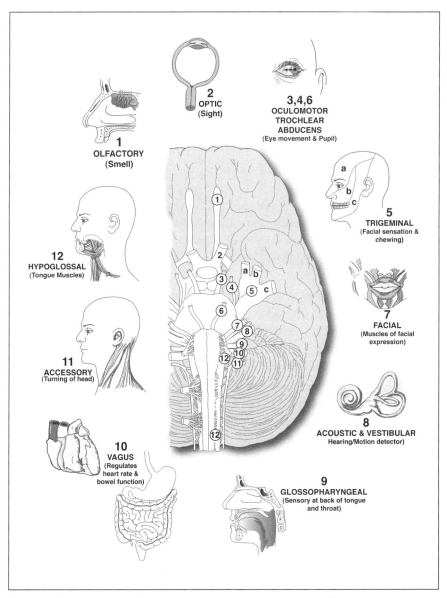

Figure 2.3 The brainstem and cranial nerves, where particular constellations of symptoms in a small warning stroke (TIA) point to reduced blood flow in specific locations

Strokes Due to Neck Injury

A special cause of stroke that is more common in young people is dissection of the arteries: the inner lining of an artery peels off and rolls up, and either can block the artery or can be a place where clots form and then break off and embolize downstream.

Dissection of an artery may be spontaneous, or it may be related to injury. The vertebral arteries, which run up through channels in the bones of the neck, are particularly vulnerable at the top of the neck, where they make a sharp turn and go up through the hole at the base of the skull through which the spinal cord connects to the brainstem (see Figure 2.4). At that point they are susceptible to injury in car crashes or through chiropractic manipulation. Even minor neck injuries sustained in yoga or swimming or when extending one's neck over the edge of a hairdressser's sink (5) have led to these strokes.

Although strokes due to chiropractic manipulation are perhaps more publicized and seldom go unrecognized by physicians, those that result from car accidents, in my experience, are not only more common (4) but also seldom diagnosed. If you are in a car accident or undergo a neck manipulation and then have symptoms that suggest loss of blood flow to the back of the brain (vertebrobasilar ischemia), such as vertigo, flashing lights in the vision, loss of vision, loss of consciousness, numbness around the mouth or on both sides of the body, or periods of amnesia, you may be having TIAs due to injury to your vertebral arteries. The period between the neck injury and the TIA or stroke can be days, weeks, months, or even, in rare cases, years.

Chiropractors say that strokes from neck manipulation are very rare, about one in a million manipulations. Most stroke experts see so many of these strokes (we now see one or two per month in our Urgent TIA Clinic) that they seem more common than that figure suggests, but perhaps there are more manipulations than we realize. In any case, even if the risk is small, to me it isn't worth taking: randomized clinical trials show that physiotherapy is as effective as chiropractic (6; 7), and without neck manipulation there is less risk of stroke. For the headaches that are often due to spasm of the neck muscles, massage therapy is also very helpful. That kind of headache

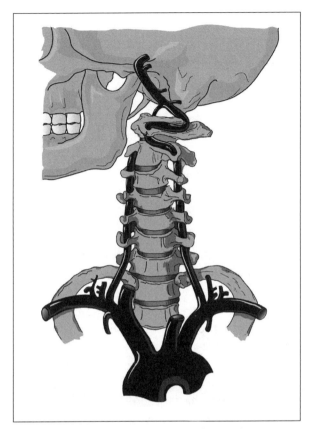

Figure 2.4 Vertebral arteries at the top of the neck, particularly vulnerable to strokes as the result of motor vehicle crashes or chiropractic manipulation

is particularly common in people with vertigo, because they are using their neck muscles to try to stop the world from spinning.

It should be clear from this chapter that a careful history is a key part of the detective work required to sort out what happened in a TIA. This is the first step to figuring out if there was a stroke or a TIA, and what caused it, so that the right treatment can be instituted to prevent another (possibly devastating) stroke.

3
Plaque in the Arteries (Atherosclerosis)

Although it is often called "hardening of the arteries" and sometimes "arteriosclerosis," I think the best name for the condition that causes heart attacks and most strokes is *atherosclerosis*. This label reminds us that there is a lot going on in the artery wall; using this term helps keep us from oversimplifying the problem. The word comes from *sclerosis*, which means scarring, and *ather*, an ancient Greek word for gruel or porridge, because the material that makes up plaques—the lesions of an affected artery—looks like oatmeal (see Figure 3.1). It is grungy, yellowish, and crumbly, with cholesterol crystals in it. It can induce clotting of the blood or can break off and embolize downstream, where it blocks branches and stops the flow of blood to whatever part of the brain, foot, bowel, kidney, or heart the branches supply.

Most people imagine that an atherosclerotic plaque is a deposit of cholesterol and fat in the artery wall, like a collection of egg yolk and butter fat that has simply been left there from excess fat in the blood. It is actually more like scar tissue in the artery wall, as we will see. Plaque is made up of inflammatory cells, fibrous tissue and smooth muscle cells that grow into the artery lining where it is injured, much like scar tissue. Some of the cells become swollen with cholesterol that they have taken up and stored.

To understand plaque and its role in stroke—as well as how to combat plaque—one first needs some understanding of arteries and of the several elegant systems that keep blood flowing freely through them.

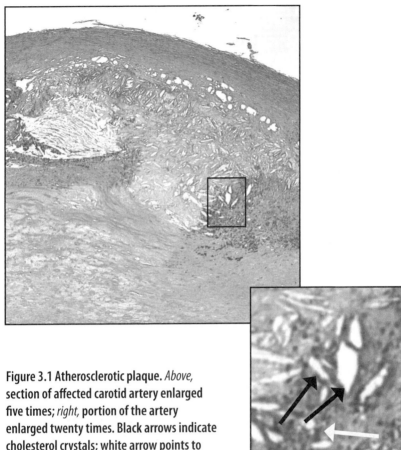

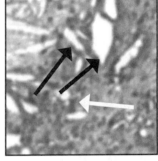

Figure 3.1 Atherosclerotic plaque. *Above,* section of affected carotid artery enlarged five times; *right,* portion of the artery enlarged twenty times. Black arrows indicate cholesterol crystals; white arrow points to inflammatory cells. *Courtesy of Dr. Robert Hammond.*

The Elegant Balance of the Artery Lining

All arteries have three layers: inner (the intima), middle (the media), and outer (the adventitia). The inner layer of each artery is covered by protective cells, which make up the endothelium; there are so many miles of arteries that the endothelium is the equivalent of a large organ, such as the liver, in size. (To help you comprehend the territory that arteries cover, a pound of fat contains about three miles of arteries and their branches.)

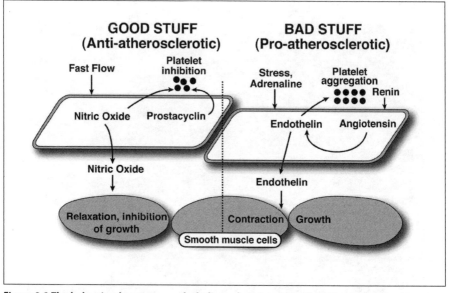

Figure 3.2 The balancing hormones endothelin and nitric oxide adjust the size of the artery to the rate of blood flow. They also affect clotting on the surface, and affect growth in the wall.

The Artery Lining: A Balancing Act

The cells of the endothelium—that is, the lining of arteries—make chemicals such as nitric oxide, which cause the artery to dilate and interfere with blood clotting, and endothelin, which promotes blood clotting and constriction of the arteries. These hormones, in a sense, maintain a balance that adjusts the size of the artery to the rate of blood flow. Their complementarity is so striking that they have been called the yin and yang of the artery wall (Figure 3.2).

In another balancing act, the endothelial cells make a second type of chemical (prostacycline) that dilates arteries and inhibits clotting (clumping of the blood platelets), while platelets themselves make and release a chemical (thromboxane) that promotes clotting and constriction of arteries. Because aspirin and drugs for arthritis block the formation of thromboxane and prostacycline, this balance becomes important in discussing doses of aspirin and the adverse effects of drugs for arthritis (8); these issues are discussed in a later chapter.

Other Protective Regulators

At the same time, the brain, spinal cord, and nerves send signals to the heart, arteries, and veins that regulate blood flow to meet the needs of the body. The heart reacts by speeding up or slowing down; the arteries and veins, by dilating or constricting.

Thus, several elegant systems keep in balance the flow of the blood and the state of the arteries, to optimize the blood flow to tissues such as the brain, and to minimize the damage to the arteriesfrom the pressure and flow of blood.

Injuries to the Artery Lining

Over the long lifespan that human beings now enjoy, these systems of elegant symmetry cannot totally prevent injury to the artery lining, or endoelium, especially where the arteries bend and branch and where disturbances occur in the blood flow.

In the normal pattern, the fastest blood flow is in the middle of the artery, and the slowest is along the artery wall, which means the artery lining is usually well protected. Disturbances in blood flow, including heartbeats, disrupt this pattern. In a year, your heart will beat, and the artery lining will be exposed to flow disturbances, about thirty to forty million times. Each beat produces a surge of pressure and flow in the arteries. In some parts of the body, the blood pulls away from the artery wall on the inside of a bend and runs into the artery wall on the outside of the bend, just like a river.

These flow disturbances interact with the hormones produced by the cells in the artery lining that regulate both artery diameter and the function of blood platelets. Along with the red blood cells and white cells, platelets—essentially packages of hormones and clotting proteins—normally travel in the fastest-moving blood in the middle of the artery. But flow disturbances can smash the platelets against an artery wall or form a lesion in that wall, that is, a rough atherosclerotic plaque. This is not good news for the flow of blood.

Bruised platelets release their hormones, not only triggering clumps of platelets that can embolize downstream to block branches but also causing the artery to constrict, which tends to disturb blood flow even further. (This is a likely cause of unstable angina, leading to chest pain at rest for individuals who previously experienced chest pain only when they exercised to a certain level.)

Besides releasing hormones, damaged platelets also release substances that stimulate the growth of the artery wall and cause the inner lining, the endothelium, to thicken. Damage to the endothelium—that is, injury to the lining of the artery—sets off a series of unhappy events. First, it attracts platelets and white blood cells to attach to the normally smooth endothelium. Next, it leads some white blood cells (monocytes) to migrate under the endothelium into the innermost layer of the artery itself (the intima), where they transform into macrophages—Pac-Man-type cells that gobble up cholesterol and other substances—and multiply. These macrophages accumulate cholesterol and form a fatty streak. Finally, smooth-muscle cells migrate from the middle muscular layer of the artery (the media), grow in the intima, and cause it to thicken further, forming a plaque.

The Response-to-Injury Hypothesis of Atherosclerosis

The entire process just described has been likened to the repair of an injury, similar to the healing of a cut by scar tissue: the sequence comprises endothelial injury, attachment of platelets and white blood cells, migration of macrophages into the innermost layer of an artery, proliferation of cells from the middle layer that thicken the innermost layer, and the deposit of cholesterol in those cells, forming a plaque. At this stage, a fibrous cap prevents the plaque's soft core, made up of inflammatory cells and cholesterol, from breaking through into the central passage of the artery through which blood flows (see Figure 3.3).

This "response to injury" hypothesis to account for atherosclerosis derives from the work of German pathologists in the nineteenth century, was brought forward to the twentieth century by Dr. Daria Haust with her colleague Dr. Bob More, and then was developed and expanded by Dr. Russell Ross and his colleagues. With recent refinements that take into account the importance of inflammation in the arteries, it probably explains atherosclerosis about as well as we can for now.

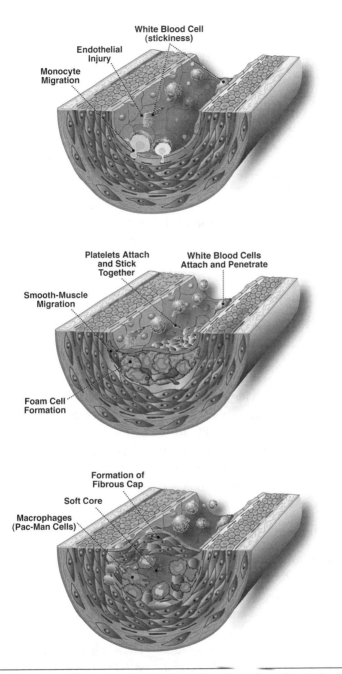

Figure 3.3 Sequence illustrating the hypothesis that plaque forms in arteries as a response to injury

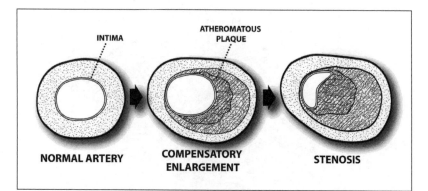

Figure 3.4 Earliest stages of atherosclerosis, as the artery enlarges to compensate for the growth of plaque. Narrowing (stenosis) probably results from plaque rupture.

The Early Stages

Although it seems logical to assume that when plaque develops in the artery wall, it should stick out into the opening in the tubelike vessel and cause it to narrow, what actually happens is that the artery enlarges to accommodate the plaque. That is, the artery compensates for the change; it gets bigger so that the flow rate along its wall remains constant. This growth is termed *compensatory enlargement* or *vascular remodeling* (see Figure 3.4).

This explains why the process can begin in the teens and progress for many years without causing trouble. (The process accelerates with age for reasons discussed in a later chapter.)

Plaque Rupture

At some point, an event occurs, such as a rupture of the plaque or a hemorrhage into the plaque. The scar formation in the plaque causes it to encroach on the artery's flow channel, which aggravates flow disturbances such as turbulence. The narrowing of arteries (stenosis) thus occurs only after a plaque ruptures.

The flow disturbances bring more platelets into contact with the wall, and more kinetic energy is transmitted to the wall. The plaque becomes inflamed; if it ruptures—that is, if the protective fibrous

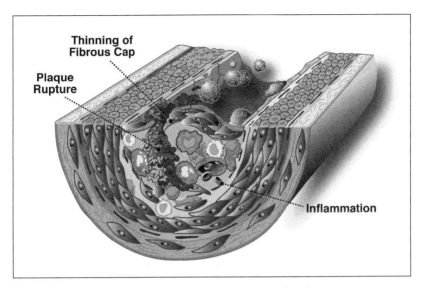

Thinning of Fibrous Cap

Plaque Rupture

Inflammation

Figure 3.5 Plaque rupture—the cause of 70–80 percent of strokes

cap of the plaque cracks open—the granular contents of the plaque may embolize downstream or provoke the local formation of clot, blocking the artery completely. In other cases, a hemorrhage into a plaque, rather than an outward rupture, causes a sudden blockage of the artery. Virtually all heart attacks, and about 70 to 80 percent of strokes, begin with a plaque rupture (see Figure 3.5).

Now that we know how to beat strokes due to high blood pressure, the main enemy is atherosclerosis. The succeeding chapters describe the weapons we have available to take into battle against it.

4
Cardiac Tests and Brain Imaging

Blood clots from the heart, or material from the heart valves, cause about 20 percent of strokes due to brain infarction—due, that is, to permanent loss of blood flow to the brain that destroys brain tissue. About 8 percent of people who have a brain infarction have recently had a heart attack (myocardial infarction) that caused the blood clot in the heart; the inner lining of the heart at the site of damage became sticky, with a tendency to form clots, which then broke off and went to the brain. Atherosclerotic plaque in the aorta, the main artery coming out of the heart, can also break off and embolize into the brain and elsewhere.

Tests to detect a heart attack include an electrocardiogram (ECG, often called EKG) and blood tests to measure enzymes or other markers in blood released from damaged heart muscle.

Strokes Caused by Blood Clots from the Heart

A cardiac (or aortic) source of emboli is suspected particularly in an individual whose stroke has no other apparent cause. Arteries in the neck appear normal on ultrasound, and an angiogram of the brain arteries (discussed later) uncovers no reason for the stroke. The heart or aorta may also be suspected as the source of emboli if a heart problem shows up in the individual's medical history or in the physical exam at the time of the stroke.

Heart Rhythm Disorders

For example, one symptom that may show up is an irregular heart rhythm, leading to the detection of a rhythm disorder called *atrial fibrillation*. Normally, the atrium or upper chamber of the heart beats in a coordinated way to propel blood down into the ventricle, the main pumping chamber of the heart. When the atrium fibrillates, it wiggles like a bag of worms in an uncoordinated way, so the blood sits around in a sort of sidesaddle called the auricle (because it's shaped like an ear); since this blood is not moving, it can form a clot, which can break off in chunks that make their way into the blood going to the brain.

Tests to detect such cardiac rhythm disturbances include an ECG, a twenty-four-hour recording of the ECG onto a tape recorder (a Holter recording), and sometimes a recording onto a loop recorder that can be worn for weeks at a time and triggered if there is an event.

Aneurysms

Another main cause of emboli from the heart is a bulge in the wall of the heart, called an *aneurysm*. This is similar to a bulge on the wall of a tire; it is an area of scar tissue resulting usually from a previous heart attack. The damaged part of the muscle has been replaced by a scar that does not beat, and that tends to become a larger bulge with time. The blood in the aneurysm isn't moving properly, so it tends to clot and then has the potential to embolize. An aneurysm shows up on an echocardiogram, which is an ultrasound scan of the heart.

Blood Circulation and Filtering

The heart has an electrical system for triggering contraction of its various chambers and parts in a coordinated way, so that the blood flows smoothly around a circuit (see Figure 4.1). The blood runs from the large veins into the upper chamber, or atrium, on the right side of the heart; the right atrium propels the blood into the right ventricle, the main pumping chamber; and the right ventricle pumps blood into the lung arteries via the large pulmonary artery. The lung

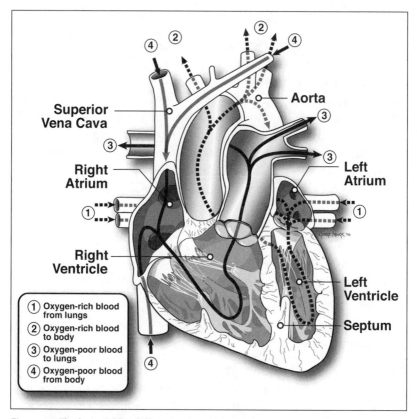

Figure 4.1 The heart's blood-flow circuit, which carries oxygen-rich blood from the lungs to the body and returns oxygen-poor blood back to the lungs

arteries branch into smaller and smaller arteries, and then finally into tiny capillaries, which act as very fine filters.

The capillaries then empty into even tinier venules, which join together into larger and larger veins, which then empty into the left atrium of the heart (see Figure 4.2). The left atrium propels blood into the heart's left ventricle, which then pumps blood under higher pressure into the aorta (the main artery out of the heart), which divides into branches, including the arteries to the arms and brain, then turns to run down into the abdomen toward the legs.

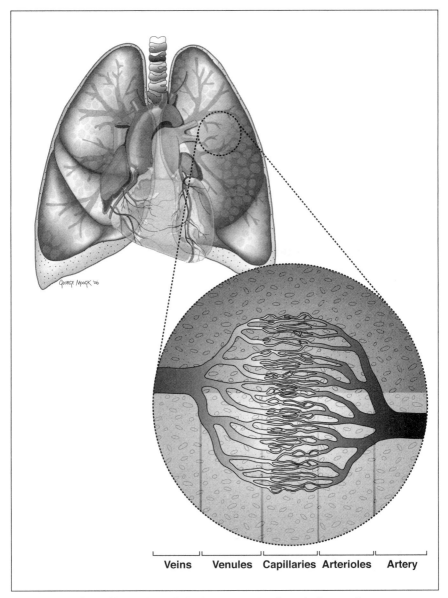

Figure 4.2 The flow of blood through the lungs, entering from the large pulmonary artery, traveling through the lungs' arteries, capillaries, and venules, and exiting into the heart's left atrium

Blockages of the Lung Artery (Pulmonary Emboli)

The filtering of the blood in the lungs is important, because it prevents clots that form in the large veins of the legs or the pelvis from going to the brain if they break off and travel up through the large veins to the heart and into the lung arteries. When a very large clot blocks the pulmonary artery, it is called a *pulmonary embolus*; in rare cases, these are fatal. Often these emboli are so small they go undiagnosed. If there is a problem with the branching of arteries into veins in the lung, or with the dividing partition between the chambers of the heart, clots large enough to cause trouble can embolize to the brain and cause stroke.

Abnormal Connections between Arteries and Veins in the Lung

Some people (and sometimes in families) have abnormally large arteries in the lungs that go straight into larger veins, without going through small capillaries. Such a malformed passage between an artery and a vein is called an *arteriovenous fistula*. In that circumstance, clots can go straight through the lung into the left side of the heart and then embolize into the brain or other parts of the systemic circulation. This accounts for about 2 percent of strokes in people under age twenty.

Problems in the Heart's Dividing Partitions

Some people are born with a defect (or a potential defect) in the dividing partition between the upper chambers (atria) of the heart or between the two main pumping chambers (ventricles). The holes in the partition between the atria are remnants of fetal circulation; the fetus needs to exchange blood between the two sides of the heart because its lungs are not yet expanded. At birth, with the first breath, a baby's lungs expand and blood begins to circulate as it will in the adult. An arterial connection between the pulmonary artery and aorta closes off within a day or so, and a flap normally seals up the hole in the partition dividing the two atria.

The commonest situation is when the hole fails to seal over at

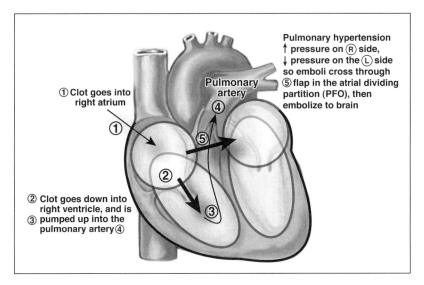

Figure 4.3 How a paradoxical embolism occurs

birth and remains covered only by a flap, which is kept closed by the higher pressure on the left side of the heart. This occurs in about 20 percent of the population, who therefore have a potential opening between the two sides of the heart that could open up if a pulmonary embolus raises the pressure on the right side of the heart.

That is, when the pulmonary artery is blocked temporarily, the blood pressure on the right side of the heart goes way up; at the same time the pressure of the blood coming back to the left side of the heart from the lungs is reduced, so the pressure on the left side goes way down. This blows open the flap over the hole in the atrial dividing partition; pieces of the clot can then cross over to the left side of the heart, from which they can embolize to the brain.

Because the blood is not supposed to go from the right side of the heart to the left, when this happens it is called a *paradoxical embolus* (Figure 4.3). Although this kind of embolus accounts for about 4–5 percent of brain infarctions, it is very often not diagnosed. It should be considered in any case where a swollen leg and/or a sudden onset of shortness of breath precede a stroke, and also in less obvious circumstances: an unexplained stroke, particularly in a young person and in anyone who has been sitting or lying around a long time so clots can form in the legs. Long transoceanic flights, prolonged sitting in front of a computer, or postoperative confinement following hip replacement or a leg fracture are typical set-ups for pulmonary emboli.

Clues to Diagnosis

There are some important clues to the diagnosis of a pulmonary embolus. It sometimes is associated with loss of consciousness at the onset of the stroke, because when the pulmonary artery is blocked temporarily, blood flow stops and the individual passes out. It is often, though not always, associated with phlebitis and a swelling of one leg due to deep vein thrombosis (clotting). It is also more likely to occur in someone with a family history of deep vein thrombosis and pulmonary emboli, because of an inherited disorder that causes excessive blood clotting. Paradoxical embolism is more common after a prolonged period of inactivity, such as a long plane or car ride or confinement after an operation that promotes the formation of thrombus in the deep veins of the legs. Also, paradoxical emboli may be provoked by straining while lifting something heavy, or during a bowel movement or delivery of a baby, because the straining increases the pressure in the right side of the heart.

Tests that demonstrate the anatomical setup for this kind of embolus include nuclear medicine scans, which will show that the lung is not filtering properly in the case of a pulmonary arteriovenous fistula, or an echocardiogram or transcranial Doppler with a "bubble test" (described later).

The key issue with all these clots from the heart is that the treatment for them is different from than for other kinds of stroke. When emboli from the heart are suspected, the treatment is with strong drugs that prevent clotting—anticoagulants.

Because using anticoagulants involves risk and inconvenience, and because missing the diagnosis of a pulmonary embolus will lead to the wrong treatment, it can be very important to determine that there is a cardiac source of emboli. Although sometimes tests don't discover the source, it is worth looking for, particularly when the stroke is otherwise unexplained.

Testing for Lung-Artery Blockage

The tests most commonly employed to detect pulmonary emboli include electrocardiograms, echocardiograms, nuclear medicine scans to assess the blood flow to the heart muscle, and occasionally cardiac and/or pulmonary angiograms. Transcranial Doppler can also be used to detect the passage of bubbles into the brain arteries.

Electrocardiogram

An electrocardiogram, or ECG, is an electrical recording from the limbs and the surface of the chest that shows the pattern of electrical activity in the heart. The ECG can detect rhythm disturbances such as atrial fibrillation, may detect the presence of an old myocardial infarction, and in some circumstances, particularly when repeated daily for several days, can detect a recent heart attack (myocardial infarction). The accuracy of this diagnosis by ECG is greatly aided by measuring enzymes or other markers from the heart released into the bloodstream when the heart muscle breaks down, such as CK (creatine phosphokinase) and troponin.

An electrocardiogram requires sticking electrodes to the limbs and the chest, and then making a recording. It is completely safe and is painless (except for the pulling of chest hair when the electrodes are removed).

Echocardiogram

An ultrasound examination called an *echocardiogram—echo*, for short—reveals the action of the heart valves, as well as the pattern of contraction of the heart muscle and areas that are not contracting, including aneurysms. Valves at the outlet of each chamber of the heart prevent the blood from going backward in the system. Sometimes problems with the valves can lead to stickiness on their surface, and to a buildup of clot or a clump of clotting protein and inflammatory cells, which may be infected.

The echo usually involves an ultrasound probe applied to the chest, with some lubricating gel to make a good contact. Sound beams are directed into the heart, and a computer analyzes the return echoes and converts them into images. The test is completely safe and harmless; it is essentially the same kind of imaging used to check out babies in the uterus.

Occasionally, if the usual echocardiogram through the chest wall is unsatisfactory, the test may require putting a tube into the esophagus (the tube that goes from the mouth to the stomach). That procedure is called a *transesophageal echocardiogram*, or TEE. This may be particularly important for detecting either aortic plaque or a defect in the atrial dividing partition. In the latter case, the method is called a *bubble test*, or *saline test*; it detects an atrial defect by mixing air with a salt solution to form tiny bubbles, injecting them into a vein, and then seeing if the bubbles pass through the partition.

Because one must swallow the ultrasound probe and the procedure takes a while, there is some discomfort with TEE and a sedative is commonly used. There is also a slight risk of aspiration pneumonia (which happens when the person vomits and then breathes the vomitus into the lungs), a serious condition. Because of that risk, if you are scheduled for a TEE, you will probably be advised not to eat or drink anything the day of the test until after you have recovered from the sedative. Fortunately the risk is very small, and if a stroke is unexplained and no other logical treatment has been identified, the increased accuracy of the diagnosis justifies it.

Holter Recording

Another method for detecting rhythm disturbances besides the ECG is the Holter recording, most often used to diagnose atrial fibrillation (AF), one of the important causes of stroke from emboli from the heart. This condition, in which clots form in the left atrium (the upper pumping chamber on the left, or systemic, side of the heart) is usually suspected because the rhythm of the pulse is very irregular. Since there is no pattern to the irregularity of rhythm, it is said to be "irregularly irregular."

In most cases atrial fibrillation can be confirmed by an ECG, but in some cases the ECG misses the diagnosis because the AF is intermittent. It probably takes less than a day of AF to form a clot that can embolize, so some strokes may be due to an episode of AF the day before, or earlier on the same day. To determine whether the person is having intermittent episodes of AF, an ECG can be recorded for twenty-four or forty-eight hours—essentially copying the ECG onto a tape recorder. A computer analyzes the tape to determine if there have been episodes of heart-rhythm disturbance, and thus episodes of AF that are not apparent to the individual experiencing them can be detected.

A Holter recording can also detect such rhythm disturbances as episodes of a very fast or very slow heart rate that might cause fainting. (You faint if your heart rate is too fast because the heart doesn't have time to fill between beats and your blood pressure drops; you faint if the heart rate is too slow because the amount of blood being pumped isn't enough to sustain brain function.) Also, the recording system can detect ECG changes during episodes when there is insufficient blood supply to the heart muscle (myocardial ischemia).

Nuclear Medicine Scanning

A nuclear medicine scan assesses how well blood is flowing to the heart muscle (myocardium) and is most useful for diagnosing coronary artery disease in individuals whose routine treadmill stress test is inconclusive, or who can't take that test.

Many people with coronary artery disease have a history of chest pain brought on by exertion and relieved by rest; others may exhibit no symptoms, and about 40 percent of myocardial infarctions are "silent"—a heart attack occurred without any chest pain or other symptoms that led to its recognition. One way to test for a suspected problem with the coronary arteries is to do a stress test: the individual walks on a treadmill while hooked up to an ECG recording, the level of exercise is gradually increased, and the ECG is observed. If there is a problem with a partial blockage of one of the arteries, it shows up as a change in the electrical pattern on the ECG, and the test is regarded as positive.

When an individual can't undergo a routine exercise stress test because of problems such as a bad hip or knee, or because of shortness of breath due to lung problems, a nuclear medicine scan can perform the same diagnosis. This scan involves injecting a small dose of a radioactive tracer into a vein while the individual's heart is speeded up either by some kind of exercise such as rotating a pedal system with the arms, or by injection of a drug such as dipyridamole. An array of detectors similar to small Geiger counters detect the arrival and disappearance of the radioactive tracer in various regions of the heart muscle and thus image and measure the blood flow to the heart. If one of the coronary arteries is blocked or narrowed, the part of the myocardium that would normally get its blood supply from that artery fails to "light up" on the scan; in some cases this scan can also detect the abnormal movement of an aneurysm.

Although radioactivity sounds scary, one or even several scans poses no danger. The gamma radiation involved is the same kind we get every day from sunlight; the dose is about the equivalent of going to Denver for a week of skiing, or crossing the Atlantic once in an airliner (radiation levels are higher at higher altitudes).

Coronary Angiography

The definitive way, for now at least, to determine whether there is a problem with blockage of the coronary arteries is to do a radiological (X-ray) examination of the arteries, a procedure called *angiography*. This begins with putting a needle into the artery at the top of one leg. (The arteries to the legs join in the middle, in the aorta, which is the main artery leaving the heart; all the other arteries are branches of the aorta.) A thin plastic tube called a *catheter* is threaded through the needle and advanced up through the bloodstream until it reaches the top of the aorta, just where it leaves the heart. The catheter is maneuvered into the opening of each coronary artery—the first branches off the aorta, just above the aortic valve—and an injection of X-ray contrast material, or dye, is injected through the catheter to show up the artery and its branches.

The feeling of heat that once accompanied each injection is much diminished with the development of newer dyes (nonionic contrast material), which are slightly safer than the older dyes and cost about ten times more.

Under development are methods to image the coronary arteries by MRI or CT angiography that do not require a catheter to be inserted into the heart. However, because the artery narrowing often can be treated with angioplasty and stenting (in which a tube is inserted into an artery to keep the passage open), and a catheter is required for those treatment procedures, angiography will remain common.

The Risks of Testing

If you have a long drive from home to the hospital, the risk of your round-trip drive is probably not much less than the risk of most of the tests just described.

An angiogram does carry a small risk, so it shouldn't be done without a good reason. The risks include a reaction to the X-ray dye (discussed later), as well as a serious complication from an injury to one of the arteries—about a 1:1,000 risk of dying or needing an operation immediately to reopen a coronary artery blocked because the dye injection caused a peeling off or "dissection" of the artery lining.

The risk is higher if an angioplasty is done as a result of the angiogram, and a balloon is inflated to stretch open the narrow segment of the artery: probably about a 1:100 risk of needing an operation to reopen a dissected artery, and a risk of stroke due to chunks breaking off the artery wall and embolizing to the brain.

Rarely, a blood clot forms on the end of the catheter, breaks off, and embolizes to the brain or another part of the body; the risk of this complication is probably less than 1:1000.

Usually a test that carries a risk is done only if there is a reasonable chance that the result will permit treatment that will reduce the risk level that already exists. For example, individuals who have had small warning strokes (TIAs) have approximately a 30 percent risk of stroke or death within three years. In that high-risk situation, finding the cause and putting in place a course of treatment that will reduce the risk by 50 percent or more is worth taking a small chance.

Brain Imaging

I think it was Arthur Clarke, the science-fiction writer, who said that the more advanced technology becomes, the more indistinguishable it becomes from magic. We are really approaching that state with advanced imaging of the brain.

The problem with taking ordinary X-rays of the head is that the skull is so dense that it shows up very well but it also blocks the view of the brain; it's like trying to take a picture of a room from outside it with the door closed.

CT Scanning

With the invention of powerful computers, it became possible to develop software that led to a solution to the problem with ordinary brain X-rays. In computerized axial tomography, or *CAT scanning* (*CT scanning*, for short), an X-ray tube is rotated around the body; across from it a radiation detector is linked to a computer. In a sense, an X-ray slice of the brain is taken, and the density of every spot in the slice is calculated from every angle as the machine rotates around the long axis of the body.

The computer effectively cancels out the blocking effect of the bone and other structures around each spot and creates an image by plotting the density of each spot on a grid. The size of the spot is determined by the speed of the procedure and the power of the computer and software, but on average each spot, called a pixel, is about a half millimeter in diameter (about 1/64th of an inch). That level of resolution is very useful for making pictures of the brain.

Because the computer calculates the density of each spot, it is possible to compare a normal area of brain with an area nearby that has reduced density or increased density. For example, in a part of the brain where an infarction has occurred, the swelling in the damaged area causes a reduced density that looks darker; where there has been a hemorrhage, the iron in the hemoglobin in blood causes increased density, which looks lighter because it blocks the x-ray beam (see Figure 4.4).

The development of CT scanning revolutionized the management of stroke. For the first time it became possible to be sure whether a stroke was due to a hemorrhage or an infarct, and it became apparent that clinical diagnosis was wrong as often as 30 percent of the time. This is good news for stroke victims, of course, as the diagnosis guides the treatment, and an inaccurate diagnosis leads to incorrect treatment. For example, as we have seen, if a blood clot from the heart is suspected, the treatment is strong anticlotting or antico-agulant drugs; when a stroke is due to a hemorrhage, with bleeding

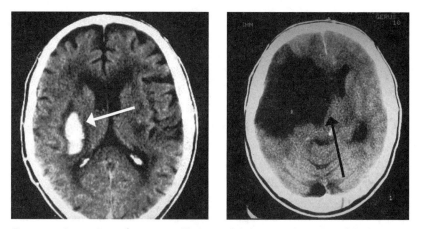

Figure 4.4 Comparison of areas on a CT scan. *Left (white arrow),* an area of the brain that is more dense on CT because of a hemorrhage; *right (black arrow),* an area of the brain that is less dense on CT because it has permanently lost its blood supply (an infarction). *Courtesy of Dr. David Pelz.*

into the brain from a ruptured artery, anticoagulants may make the situation worse.

There is very little risk from a single CT scan. The only risk is associated with the amount of radiation, which is equivalent to several chest X-rays, a concern only for pregnant women or for individuals who have repeated multiple X-ray exposures.

One problem with CT scanning is that detecting infarction depends on the swelling of the brain tissue in the area of infarction; this means that a CT scan done immediately after the event, before swelling occurs, may look normal.

MRI Scanning

It is becoming apparent that magnetic resonance imaging (MRI) scanning will significantly advance the evaluation of stroke. Unlike CT scanning, this procedure doesn't use X-rays and so carries no risk from radiation. Further, in diagnosing the cause of strokes, MRI pictures, compared to a CT scan, not only are of a finer resolution but also show changes earlier, which may make a difference in the treatment prescribed.

MRI scanning relies on the natural signals, similar to radio waves, that every atom in the body emits in response to spinning during changes in a magnetic field.

For this procedure, the individual enters a tube surrounded by a powerful electromagnet, and the magnet is switched on and off rapidly and repeatedly. What happens is that the atoms in the body line up in the magnetic field when it switches on, like iron filings near a magnet, and then they spin back into place when it switches off. As they spin back, they emit waves similar to radio waves, and the computer detects their location in a way similar to radio detection equipment you see in spy movies.

A computer maps the location and signal intensity of each spot in a way similar to the mapping of X-ray density on the CT scan. It reconstructs a picture of the brain (and other tissues), providing information that can be used to diagnose the location and type of stroke (infarct or hemorrhage) (see Figure 4.5).

There is no known risk from exposure to the magnetic field; indeed we all live in a large magnetic field, that of the earth. There is a very small risk of serious injury if a metallic object (such as keys, or a tool left behind by a technician) is attracted by the magnet so fast that it may penetrate the body. This is extremely rare, because every MRI team takes stringent precautions to prevent it.

In addition to making pictures of the brain in MRI scans, the computer can detect arteries, because the movement of the blood through them distorts the magnetic signal.

MRA

A procedure called *magnetic resonance angiography,* or MRA, which involves injecting dye (contrast material, such as gadolinium), produces even better pictures of the arteries than do MRI scans. In most centers MRA is not quite as accurate as angiography for seeing small structures such as small aneurysms, but the technology is improving.

This procedure is probably quite effective for excluding the existence of large cerebral aneurysms in individuals who are being screened because of a family history of brain hemorrhages due to brain aneurysms; it may also be adequate to evaluate whether individuals with strokes in the arteries to the back of the brain (the

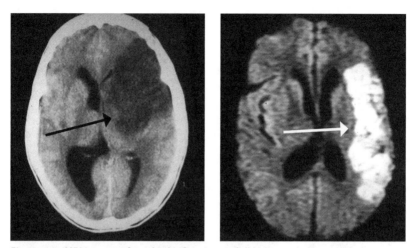

Figure 4.5   MRI images of cerebral infarction. *Left (black arrow)*, a large infarction shows up as a dark area; *right (white arrow)*, swelling shows up as a white area in a diffusion-weighted scan, particularly good for early detection of infarction. *Courtesy of Dr. David Pelz.*

vertebrobasilar system, as discussed in Chapter 2) need treatment with anticoagulants. The advantage of this finding is that it may make angiography unnecessary. (In Figure 4.6, which compares an MRA image and an angiogram, another high-tech method, digital subtraction angiography—DSA—has been used to subtract the skull and jaw bones from the angiogram image.)

NEW DEVELOPMENTS IN MRI

Imaging scientists are developing methods that combine imaging and spectroscopy that make it possible to assess the metabolism of the brain in different regions, and even to assess brain function. For example, if you think of names for colors, a different part of your brain lights up than when you think of names for animals. When violin music is played, in non-violinists the parts of the brain related to listening, hearing, and music light up; in right-handed violinists, violin music lights up not only those parts of the brain but also the parts that control the fingers of the left hand, because the violinists are imagining the fingering!

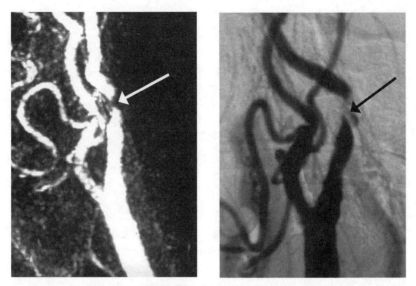

Figure 4.6 Comparison of images from an MRA and an ordinary angiogram. *Left (white arrow)*, an MRA shows a severe narrowing of the carotid artery; *right (black arrow)*, a regular angiogram shows the same artery. *Courtesy of Dr. David Pelz.*

Artery Imaging: Doppler Ultrasound

Ultrasound uses sound waves to measure the degree of narrowing of the arteries by measuring how fast the blood is moving through them. Ultrasound scanners are considered completely safe; indeed, obstetrical ultrasound is routinely used to check the condition of fetuses in the womb.

The Doppler Effect

If you are standing on a street corner when a car goes by honking its horn, you hear a higher pitch as the car comes toward you than when it goes away. The pitch of the horn doesn't actually change, but the car's movement past you changes its apparent pitch. The reason is that the sound waves arrive at your ears closer together as the car gets closer to you so the apparent pitch is higher, because the closer together sound waves are, the higher-pitched the sound; the sound waves are farther apart as the car gets farther away, so the pitch sounds lower.

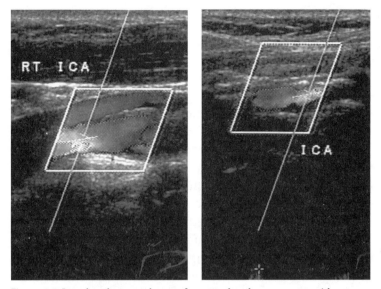

Figure 4.7 Doppler ultrasound scan of a normal and a narrow carotid artery. Blood has to go faster to get through a narrow artery. The left panel shows a normal internal carotid artery; the blood velocity is 41.4 cm/second. The right panel shows a carotid artery which has a narrowing of approximately 60%, with an increased blood velocity of 198.1 cm/second

This apparent shift due to movement is named after Christian Andreas Doppler, who first noticed the effect in the color of light waves emitted by stars. Beginning in the 1960s, scientists used the Doppler shift of ultrasound to reflect sound waves off red blood cells: the change in pitch of the reflected sound indicated how fast the blood was moving.

The significance of ultrasound for diagnosing narrowed arteries is this: if an artery is narrow, the blood has to speed up to get through the narrowing, so high-velocity signals on an ultrasound represent narrowing. Figure 4.7 compares a normal artery and a narrow artery in which the blood is faster, similar to the rapids in a river, speeding up to get through the narrowing.

The ultrasound devices that are now in general use can also make pictures of the artery by analyzing the reflections of the sound wave, like echoes, from the artery wall. These duplex scanners use both imaging and Doppler flow information for diagnoses.

Plaque Measurement

Since about 1990 it has been possible via ultrasound to see the plaque in the artery wall.

2-D PLAQUE MEASUREMENT

As far as I know, measurement of carotid plaque began in our laboratory. Some years ago, I was interested not only in measuring the speed of the blood to calculate the degree of arterial narrowing but also in what was happening in the wall of the artery. I asked our ultrasound technologists to make drawings of the arteries, showing the location and size of plaques, so we could compare from year to year and see if a patient's arteries were getting better or worse. One day in 1992, I asked our wonderful ultrasound technologist, Maria DiCicco, RVT (registered vascular technologist), how I could tell if she was making the drawings in a way that was consistent from one year to the next. Her reply was: "Well, Dr. Spence, there is software in the machine that would let me make measurements of the plaques, if you want them." So that was the beginning of plaque measurement. She began to measure the atherosclerotic plaque in carotid arteries by tracing around the image of the plaque with a cursor on the screen of the ultrasound machine. A computer in the machine then prints out the area of the plaque in two dimensions (see Figure 4.8). We have used such 2-D measurements of plaque area in our lab since 1992 to study the effects of stress and other new risk factors, and the effects of treatments such as vitamins or cholesterol-lowering drugs.

Plaque measurements are very useful, because they not only identify who is at high risk but also provide feedback on the effectiveness of treatment.

If all the plaques are measured, and the total area of plaque is added up, this gives very powerful information about both risk and response to therapy. Individuals with a lot of plaque have a higher risk of stroke, death, and heart attack: those in the top quartile of plaque have a five-year risk that is 3.4 times higher than those in the bottom quartile, even after adjusting for all the traditional risk factors (11). Furthermore, those whose plaques increase in the first year despite treatment of the traditional risk factors have twice the risk of those with stable plaque or regression. For those individuals, physicians need to try harder. Tests can investigate newer risk

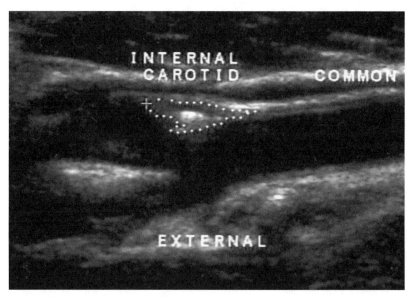

Figure 4.8 2-D measurement of carotid plaque area, which shows arterial plaque of 0.18 cm². This is a method both for evaluating the risk of heart attacks and strokes and for evaluating whether therapy is working. *Courtesy of Maria DiCicco, RVT.*

factors such as homocysteine (an amino acid that increases clotting and irritates the lining of blood vessels), lipoprotein (a), borderline hypothyroidism, borderline B_{12} deficiency (12), and so on. In cases where the plaque is progressing despite good control of all known or suspected risk factors, the physician needs to try to figure out what is causing the problem. In families that are large enough, it is now possible to do genetic testing to find the cause, which will eventually lead to the appropriate treatment.

3-D PLAQUE VOLUME

The latest development in this field is the ability to measure plaque volume in three dimensions (3-D) using ultrasound. A fast computer that can capture and store images rapidly can in essence store data from a rectangular block of tissue in the neck, including the carotid arteries, in a couple of minutes. A technician can then use the computer to look at cross-sectional slices of the artery, measuring plaque in each slice, as for 2-D scans. The difference is that each slice has thickness (this can be set from one to four millimeters), so the computer can add up the slices like a stack of salami pieces to compute the volume of the plaque. This method is clearly the best available for studying a number of situations, including the effects of interventions such as vitamins or cholesterol-lowering drugs, and will soon revolutionize the study of arteries (13).

It is now possible to measure the 3-D volume of plaques in the carotid arteries and to map the surface roughness, which is related to the amount of ulceration of the artery lining (14). Figure 4.9 shows plaque measurements and displays mapping of plaque surface roughness in the same carotid artery shown in Figure 4.8.

X-Rays of Brain Arteries (Cerebral Angiography)

Although often replaced now with a combination of ultrasound and MRA, angiography—X-ray examination of the arteries—is still necessary in some cases. It is the best way to find a brain aneurysm or arteriovenous malformation (AVM, a growth of abnormal blood vessels in the brain, similar to a birthmark) and to plan surgery for these conditions; and angiography is sometimes necessary to see inflammation of the arteries (vasculitis).

Sometimes an angiogram is needed for treatment. For the carotid arteries, and sometimes even for the arteries inside the head, angioplasty (the insertion of a catheter and then of a balloon, inflated to stretch open the narrow segment of the artery) and stenting (insertion of a tube to keep the passage open) are now being done in selected cases. The clot-buster tPA (tissue plasminogen activator) can be injected through a catheter into the brain arteries in some cases; aneurysms can be blocked with coils of platinum that cause them to fill with thrombus so they won't rupture; and AVMs can sometimes be closed by injecting material similar to superglue.

The procedure for cerebral angiography is similar to that described for coronary angiography. A needle is inserted into a large artery, usually in the leg; a thin plastic catheter is advanced through the bloodstream to where the brain arteries branch off the aorta; and the catheter is advanced into the origin of the artery. Contrast material—dye—is injected into the artery, and a picture is made of the artery and its branches.

With new computerized scanners, measurements can be taken

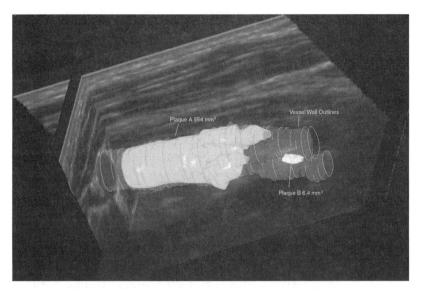

Figure 4.9   3-D measurement of plaque volume by tracing each slice (1mm apart), the best method for studying the effects of various interventions such as vitamins or cholesterol-lowering drugs. *Right,* plaque measuring 6.4 mm³; *left,* 554 mm³. *Courtesy of Dr. Aaron Fenster and Christopher Blake.*

from the screen, and the images are stored in a computer for analysis; the computer prints some representative images, often on film that looks like X-ray film. The significant advantages of the new digital angiography include a great reduction in the amount of dye needed, and therefore in the risk of the procedure.

Risks

As for coronary angiography, the risks of cerebral angiography include reactions to the dye and injury to the arteries by the needle or the catheter. The risk of dying from a bad reaction to the dye is approximately 1:40,000. There is some risk of damage to the kidneys and of heart failure, which is lessened by the reduced dose of dye when digital imaging methods are used. (Because the contrast material is denser than blood, it puts a strain on the heart similar to that caused by injecting a stronger than normal solution of salt. Kidney damage may be caused by the dye itself, but in many cases the problem seems to be the cholesterol crystals and debris from atherosclerotic plaque in the aorta that embolize into the kidney.)

Reaction to X-ray Dye

An important issue is the notion of "allergic reactions" to X-ray dye or contrast material. Although the reaction appears similar to an allergic reaction—hives, and sometimes difficulty with breathing and a severe drop in blood pressure—it is virtually never caused by a true allergy, but by a direct known effect of the contrast material on the release of histamine, an agent that dilates blood vessels.

Histamine is also released in allergic reactions, so the reaction to X-ray dye can look very similar. The reason it is important to recognize the difference is that true allergies are much more dangerous. People who have had one histamine-release reaction from X-ray dye seldom experience another, and the reaction can be virtually eliminated by antihistamine drugs and large doses of drugs similar to cortisone.

Unfortunately, there is a lot of misunderstanding about this issue, and people often believe that if they have had a previous reaction, they must never have X-ray dye again, or they will die. This is not true. If you are concerned because you have had a reaction, you should inform the radiologist so that precautions such as antihistamine and steroids (e.g., Prednisone) can be used. If you need an angiogram for a good reason, a previous dye reaction is not a compelling reason to avoid it.

A New Approach: Ultrasound-Based Management of Arteries

In the past few years, I have used a different approach in my prevention clinics to manage bad artery problems (15).

Rather than treat just the risk factors, such as high blood pressure and high cholesterol, we follow up to make sure that what we are doing is working. In most cases, we expect the arteries to be improving when the individual quits smoking, reduces intake of cholesterol and saturated fat, controls the blood pressure, and reduces the serum cholesterol to the target level—an LDL below 2 mmol/L (2 millimoles per liter) or 77 mg/dl (77 milligrams per deciliter).

What we are looking at is not just the degree of narrowing (stenosis), which is what most ultrasound labs reported. We follow the amount of plaque in the arteries, and we expect to see regression if all the usual risk factors are controlled.

When the plaques are getting bigger despite good results with the risk factors, we know we have to try harder; this may mean that the person who hasn't quit smoking may be motivated to do so, or we may need to measure the plasma homocysteine or lipoprotein (a) to determine whether we need to try a different treatment. In this way we have learned in the past few years that borderline low thyroid function and borderline low levels of vitamin B_{12} are two more easily treatable causes of worsening of the arteries. The search for new treatable factors continues.

In some cases, no known risk factor is present, and in that situation we are starting to do genetic research to find the cause.

This approach has begun to catch on elsewhere; it is used by Dr. Robert Brook and his colleagues in Ann Arbor, Michigan, and by Dr. Michel Romanens in Lausanne, Switzerland. I expect that it will become a standard way of assessing treatment of arteries. To me, trying to treat arteries without measuring plaque would be like trying to treat hypertension without measuring blood pressure.

The Bottom Line

The advances in medical imaging have revolutionized stroke prevention. If your doctor recommends that tests be done, the balance of risks is likely in favor of doing them. The risk of angiography is warranted if the reason is to plan carotid surgery (endarterectomy), to look for inflammation of the arteries (vasculitis), or to look for and treat the cause of a hemorrhage, such as an aneurysm or arteriovenous malformation. There are essentially no serious medical risks from CT scanning, magnetic resonance scanning, or ultrasound.

5

Carotid Surgery and Stenting

Medical treatment can prevent only some kinds of strokes. For example, antiplatelet agents such as ASA (aspirin) can prevent strokes due to clumps of platelets that stick to the artery wall and then break off and go through the bloodstream to the brain, and anticoagulants such as heparin and warfarin can prevent strokes due to blood clots in the heart or in the leg arteries.

A high proportion of strokes, though, are caused by plaque rupture and obstruction of arteries, or by chunks of the artery wall that break off and travel downstream in the blood until they reach a branch that is too small to get through; they stick there and block the artery.

It is increasingly clear that unstable plaque in the artery wall is the cause of most arterial events; the clot (thrombus) that forms in the arteries of the heart is the result of a crack or rupture of a plaque in the coronary arteries. To prevent strokes due to embolization of chunks of plaque, it is necessary either to remove the plaque, or to cover it.

What can be done depends largely on where the problem is. If the emboli in the brain are coming from the carotid artery (see Figure 2.1a), it is possible to remove the plaque surgically.

Cleaning Out the Carotid Artery Lining

An endarterectomy is an operation in which a surgeon removes the inner lining of an artery, along with the plaque attached to it. In the case of blockage in the carotid artery, the surgeon makes an incision along the length of the neck, exposing the artery, and clamps the artery above and below the area that needs to be cleaned out. The artery is then opened lengthwise, and the inner lining and plaque are removed. The artery is then sewn closed, the clamps removed, and the skin sutured.

Where to Have the Surgery

Most surgical teams think a general anesthetic is the safest choice because the deep anesthetic reduces brain metabolism (sort of like putting a computer into hibernation mode to save the battery). In that state the brain is less likely to be damaged by the reduced blood flow when the artery is clamped.

Some teams choose a local anesthetic because the patient can tell them if the brain isn't working with the artery clamped, and then a shunt can be put in to bypass the clamp. Some teams routinely put in a shunt—the teams who don't believe that putting the shunt in may cause chunks to break off and increase the risk of stroke.

The "right" anesthetic approach isn't clear, as the evidence indicates that all these methods are equally effective. What is clear, though, is that some medical centers are better than others, and it wise to have a carotid endarterectomy performed in a center where such operations are routine, with a complication rate, established by audit, of 3 percent or less. This surgery should be done by experts with lots of practice, and if a surgeon claims a complication rate of zero, you should assume the complication rate has not been audited and find another surgeon.

Who Should Have the Surgery

The place of carotid endarterectomy is still controversial. Until 1991, nobody knew whether this operation produced better results than medical therapy, even though the surgery had been done in about a million individuals. In general, surgeons believed that the operation was beneficial, and neurologists had some doubts.

CAROTID ARTERY NARROWING
WITH WARNING SYMPTOMS OF STROKE

The issue was settled by the North American Symptomatic Carotid Endarterectomy Trial (NASCET), a clinical research project in which I participated. The study was funded by the National Institutes of Health (NIH) in Washington and was coordinated from the place I work—the Robarts Research Institute in London, Canada. The principal investigator was my teacher, Dr. H.J.M. Barnett. About a hundred centers around the world (eighty in the United States, fourteen in Canada, and a few others) enrolled individuals with symptoms and narrowing of the carotid arteries in a randomized clinical trial: half had surgery, and half did not. Both groups received the best medical therapy, including aspirin (ASA), blood-pressure control, treatment of cholesterol, and smoking-cessation advice.

For individuals with severe narrowing of the carotid arteries and symptoms, the benefit was so clear that the study was stopped after two years, when only 691 individuals had been enrolled. In persons with narrowing of 70 percent or more, stroke and death were reduced from 26 percent to 9 percent over two years; in other words, with surgery, they were nearly three times better off. (Most of the 9 percent risk was the risk of delayed heart attacks or death because individuals with bad carotid arteries have bad arteries elsewhere. The actual risk at the time of surgery was a 1 percent risk of death, and a 1 percent risk of a severe stroke, with a 4 percent risk of lesser complications.)

Another large clinical trial in Europe produced similar results; there is no longer any controversy about whether individuals with symptoms and severe narrowing of arteries should have surgery: if possible, they should. Only persons with a very high operative risk should not. For them, the possibility of angioplasty is being considered, as I discuss further on.

This trial shows the power of clinical research: only 691 individuals supplied the answer that was not clear after hundreds of thousands of endarterectomies done on a case-by-case basis, outside clinical trials!

In persons with less severe narrowing of the arteries, the benefit of surgery is much less. It is now clear that there is no benefit from surgery in individuals with narrowing less than 50 percent; with narrowing between 50 percent and 70 percent, the benefits depend on other risk factors such as ulceration of the artery, the specific symptoms (ocular vs. hemispheric), sex, and associated conditions such as diabetes.

CAROTID ARTERY NARROWING WITHOUT SYMPTOMS

Several clinical trials have addressed the issue of whether people with narrowing of the carotid arteries and no symptoms should have surgery. This issue is still controversial.

The first major study was the Asymptomatic Carotid Artery Surgery (ACAS) trial (16), also a multicenter North American trial funded by the NIH and also stopped early because the benefit of surgery seemed clear. The problem is that the benefit could only be shown because the centers participating in the study had an unusually low complication rate of surgery, the benefit was much smaller than it is for symptomatic individuals, so it is a near thing.

In ACAS, the five-year risk, projected from figures available after a shorter term, was estimated to be 11 percent without surgery versus 5 percent with surgery. This amounts to a 1 percent benefit per year, and the risk of surgery was about 3 percent, so you have to wait a few years to see a difference. Even though the relative risk reduction is 50 percent, the absolute risk reduction is only 6 percent. This means that in centers with a 3 percent surgical risk, you are slightly better off with surgery; however, the average U.S. hospital has a complication rate of about 4–6 percent, so in the average hospital you are actually no better off with surgery. More recently the European study (Asymptomatic Carotid Artery Surgery Trial, or ACAST) showed virtually identical results to ACAS: a reduction in risk from 12 percent to 6 percent, predicated on a very low surgical risk of only 3 percent.

A key question is, What is the risk of waiting and using aggressive medical therapy? It turns out that with new powerful drugs for

Table 5.1. Symptomatic vs. Asymptomatic Severe Carotid Stenosis: The number of patients who need to be treated with surgery (carotid endarterectomy) to prevent 1 stroke in 2 years

Symptomatic narrowing of the carotid artery >70%	1 patient in 6
Symptomatic moderate narrowing 50-70%	1 patient in 15
Asymptomatic narrowing >60%	1 patient in 67

Source: Adapted from Barnett HJ. Carotid endarterectomy. Lancet 2004 May 8; 363(9420):1486-87.

treating cholesterol, new and better antiplatelet agents, and vitamin treatment for high blood levels of homocysteine, medical treatment today is better than it was during the ACAS trial. The risk of the first stroke being a bad one is only 10 percent; in most cases a small warning stroke, or TIA (transient ischemic attack, that is, a temporary loss of blood flow to the brain because of a blocked artery), will lead to an endarterectomy.

Asymptomatic Individuals: Choosing Treatment

Without any other information, if I had asymptomatic narrowing of my carotid arteries, I would opt for intensive medical treatment and watchful waiting. But there are some clues that can point toward individuals for whom surgery (endarterectomy) offers greater benefit than does waiting.

The real challenge for the physician is figuring out which individuals at higher risk should have surgery. For now, there are probably three situations in which an operation might be beneficial: individuals with complete blockage of the opposite carotid artery; individuals in whom the artery surface is irregular, with an appearance of an ulcer; and individuals with asymptomatic microemboli.

Patients with a complete blockage (occlusion) of the opposite carotid artery are at higher risk of stroke and so may benefit from endarterectomy. (This is a tricky choice, though, because these individuals also have a higher risk from surgery.)

Patients in whom the artery surface is irregular, with what looks on the angiogram (or, more probably, 3-D ultrasound) like an ulcer, are at higher risk and are likely to benefit from surgery. In these cases, two new areas of research are likely to give us better answers in the next few years. One is imaging of the carotid plaques to determine which ones are more likely to be unstable. (Plaques that have a soft liquid lipid center and a thin fibrous cap are thought to be more likely to rupture; plaques that are inflamed or irregular may also pose a higher risk than homogeneous plaques.)

The second area of active research is the basis for the final group of individuals with asymptomatic carotid artery narrowing who are at higher risk and more likely to benefit from surgery: those with microemboli downstream in the brain arteries. These can be detected by transcranial Doppler, a procedure in which ultrasound probes are clamped to the side of the head and focused on the main artery to the cerebral hemisphere, the middle cerebral artery.

We have recently found that among 319 individuals with asymptomatic narrowing of the carotid arteries, 10 percent had microemboli on the transcranial Doppler study, meaning that they had unstable plaque. (In individuals with symptomatic severe narrowing of the carotid arteries, ultrasound detects an average of six asymptomatic microemboli per hour; these go away after endarterectomy.) Over the first year of follow-up in our study, the risk of stroke for the individuals with asymptomatic narrowing of the carotid arteries was 15.6 percent for those with emboli versus 1 percent for those without emboli (17). Among those who had no emboli at baseline, only 1.8 percent developed microemboli a year later. This means that persons without emboli cannot, on average, benefit from either stenting (holding the artery open with an expanding sleeve) or endarterectomy; at most centers, the risks are about 5 percent for stenting, and about 4 percent for endarterectomy.

If you have asymptomatic narrowing of a carotid artery, and your doctor recommends surgery (endarterectomy) or stenting, I recommend that you insist on a transcranial Doppler embolus-detection study. If an hour of monitoring on two occasions a week apart fails to detect two or more emboli, you will be better off choosing intensive medical therapy; put off your surgery or stenting until symptoms develop, or until microemboli develop. (It would be reasonable to have this test on an annual basis.)

Bypass Surgery

Two types of bypass surgery related to arterial blockage are a bypass from an artery on the surface of the brain to an artery on the outside of the skull (extracranial-to-intracranial bypass) and a bypass between the arteries to the arms in the case of subclavian steal—"subclavian" because these arteries lie beneath the clavicle, or collarbone.

Extracranial to Intracranial Bypass

In the 1980s, advances in microsurgery led to a new operation for individuals with complete blockage of the carotid artery, an extracranial-to-intracranial (EC-IC) bypass. The surgeon opened up a hole in the skull, like a window, and connected an artery on the surface of the brain to an artery on the outside of the skull. But this procedure was generally discontinued after a multicenter clinical trial (also led by Dr. Henry Barnett at the Robarts Research Institute) showed that, on average, individuals who underwent surgery were worse off than those who didn't.

Because there are some individuals in whom it seems likely that surgery should help, the medical community is now looking at the issue of EC-IC bypass again, with newer techniques for assessing blood flow in the brain. Positron emission tomography (PET) scanning, functional magnetic resonance imaging (MRI), and new methods using CT scans are making it possible to identify individuals who are at high risk without surgery, and who may therefore benefit from it. One procedure used instead of bypass surgery (temporal-dural synangiosis) involves placing part of the temporal muscle, located at the side of the head, on the surface of the outer lining of the brain; the temporal muscle's arteries grow through to supply the brain underneath.

Subclavian Steal

The vertebral arteries, which run up through the bones at the back of the neck, are branches of the arteries to the arms (subclavian arteries). If the artery to one arm becomes blocked, the blood will go up one vertebral artery, down the other, and out into the arm with the blocked artery, "stealing" blood from the back of the brain (see Figure 5.1).

Because the blood supply to the brainstem and back of the brain is affected, typical symptoms may include vertigo, thickened speech, double vision, staggering, seeing flashing lights, loss of vision, and loss of consciousness. Such symptoms can be provoked by using the arm in a way that increases blood flow to the arm (and thus away

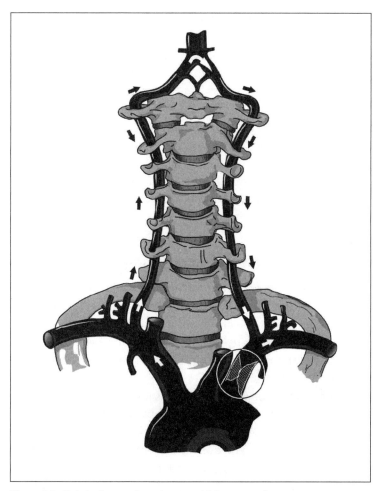

Figure 5.1 Subclavian steal syndrome, which occurs when an artery to one arm is blocked. To compensate, the artery at the back of the neck on the opposite side "steals" blood from the back of the brain and sends it down the other vertebral artery into the affected arm.

from the brain), such as sawing, hammering, hanging curtains, or reaching up to a high shelf.

For the most part, this syndrome is best managed medically. Once you understand what the problem is, you can manage the symptoms by stopping the activity in which you are using your arm, sitting or lying down, and waiting for the blood flow to return to normal.

In some cases, though, symptoms are so frequent, even with minimal use of the arm, that a bypass operation is indicated. In my opinion, it is better to do a bypass from one arm to the other (a sub-clavian-to-subclavian bypass) than a bypass from the carotid artery to the subclavian artery. The problem with the latter is that it puts all your eggs in one basket: if it goes wrong, you may have strokes in both the carotid and subclavian territories, which spells disaster. If the subclavian artery is not completely blocked, then stenting (hold-ing the artery open with an expanding sleeve) would likely be a good option.

Cleaning Out the Vertebral Artery Lining

Some people who have transient ischemic attacks (small warning strokes) in the territory of the vertebral arteries have a severe nar-rowing of the origin of the vertebral artery where it comes off the artery to the arm. A complete blockage of the artery is not usually a problem, as the vertebral artery on the other side is a backup artery that supplies the same territory.

Rarely, surgery may be required on this lesion in individuals who keep having emboli in the brain (presumably, chunks of plaque from the artery wall) despite treatment with anticlotting agents.

One procedure that can be done is an endarterectomy, which as we have seen involves removing the inner lining of an artery, along with the plaque attached to it. The operation in this case requires the surgeon to enter the subclavian artery and reach up with a little hook to turn the vertebral artery inside out, like a sock. The plaque is removed, the vertebral artery is tucked back up where it belongs, and the subclavian artery is sutured.

I suspect that with more effective drugs for cholesterol, and vita-mins for homocysteine, this surgery will become even less common. (Stenting may become a more favored option, as discussed later.)

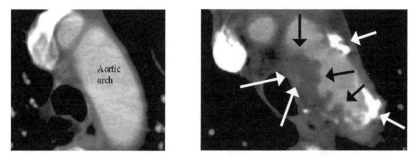

5.2 CT scan with x-ray contrast material showing plaque in the aortic arch. *Left,* a normal aortic arch, light colored because of x-ray contrast material in the bloodstream; *right,* scan indicates plaques—dark areas *(black arrows)*—and calcification, where part of the plaque has become bony *(white arrows). Courtesy of Drs. Richard Chan, Donald Lee, and Irene Gulka.*

Dealing with Aortic Plaque

With the development of better ultrasound examinations of the heart, it has become apparent that the aorta—the main artery leaving the heart—is a source of emboli to the brain. The part of the aortic arch just above the heart, before the arteries to the brain branch off, can form plaques that can become unstable and be the source of either platelet clumps or chunks of plaque.

To diagnose this condition, an echocardiograph is usually necessary; as mentioned earlier, in this procedure the individual swallows an ultrasound probe that lodges behind the heart and aorta, in the esophagus (thus, transesophageal echocardiography, or TEE). Another approach is to do a CT scan with intravenous injection of X-ray contrast material (Figure 5.2).

For the most part, the best treatment is a combination of anti-clotting agents and aggressive medical treatment of risk factors to try to stabilize the plaques. Some experts recommend anticoagulants such as warfarin and heparin.

I know of only one surgical operation undertaken to replace the aortic arch; this is terribly high-risk surgery that can't be regarded as anything but experimental for now. Another possibility might be angioplasty, as discussed next.

Angioplasty and Stenting

In the past few years there have been major advances in treating the arteries with plastic tubes inserted through a needle puncture in an artery. Usually a needle is inserted in the main artery to the leg at the upper end of the leg; then a thin plastic tube, a catheter, is inserted through the needle and advanced through the bloodstream to the artery that is in trouble.

For individuals with abnormal blood vessels or large aneurysms in the brain (structures similar to blisters on the artery wall), it is sometimes possible to inject platinum wires, and sometimes glue, through a catheter into the aneurysm or abnormal vessel to prevent future hemorrhages. Sometimes detachable balloons can be inflated in the artery or aneurysm and then left there to block it and prevent hemorrhage.

For arteries that are causing trouble because they are too narrow, a stiff-walled balloon on the tip of a catheter can be used to dilate the artery, a procedure called *angioplasty*. This method is most useful where the problem is due to reduced blood flow in the heart, leg arteries, or kidney arteries. In the brain, however, because there are so many backup arteries, the problems from blocked arteries are mainly due not to reduced blood flow but to emboli, that is, chunks of artery wall or of plaque. For that reason it seems likely that in most cases simple angioplasty will not be as useful for preventing strokes as another procedure, stenting.

In coronary and other arteries that do not stay open after a simple angioplasty to dilate them, it is necessary sometimes to place a metal frame, or stent, like a self-expanding sleeve over the balloon used in angioplasty. When the balloon is inflated, the stent opens up and holds itself in place against the artery wall, so that it stays there when the balloon is deflated (see Figure 5.3).

Because a stent in essence covers the artery wall with a mesh, preventing chunks from embolizing, a stent in the carotid artery, the vertebral area, or possibly the aorta is likely to be useful for preventing strokes. (Aortic stents would have to be huge and could likely only be put in place with an operation that involves entering the aorta with a larger catheter than could be passed through a needle.)

At present, the stents available are not perfect for the carotid

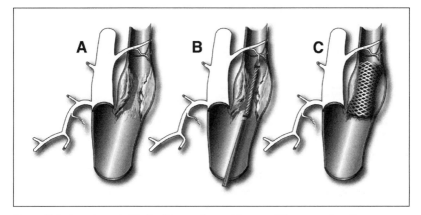

Figure 5.3 Stenting of a blocked internal carotid artery (A), a procedure for preventing strokes by inserting a metal device, a stent, over the balloon used in angioplasty (B); inflating the balloon opens the stent (C), which expands to cover the artery wall and thus prevent chunks of plaque or artery wall from breaking off and entering the bloodstream.

arteries: they can kink when you turn your neck. So far, several clinical trials have shown that angioplasty of the carotid arteries carries a much higher risk than carotid endarterectomy (cleaning out the interior artery wall) done well, and stenting carries a similar risk to endarterectomy. In my view, stenting should be used only for individuals who have a high enough risk to warrant endarterectomy; it may be the preferable procedure for individuals who are at high risk for surgery.

Based on present evidence, the risk is higher with a stent than with medical treatment in individuals with asymptomatic narrowing of the carotid arteries, with the possible exception of those in whom transcranial Doppler reveals microemboli, as discussed earlier in this chapter.

Bottom-Line Advice

If you have *symptomatic* severe narrowing of a carotid artery, you are better off with surgery than without it; the balance is about three to one in favor of surgery, if you have surgery in a very good center with an operative risk rate of about 5 percent or less.

If you have *asymptomatic* narrowing of a carotid artery without microemboli on a transcranial Doppler, you cannot benefit from either endarterectomy or stenting, because the risk of either is about five times higher than the risk of medical therapy. If someone advises endarterectomy or stenting for asymptomatic carotid stenosis, I recommend that you insist on a TCD embolus-detection study; if the doctor refuses, you should walk away quickly and go elsewhere.

If you are considering extracranial-to-intracranial bypass, I recommend that you have this surgery only in the context of a clinical trial. I say that because this procedure is experimental, and it is unwise to do experiments on one individual at a time—nothing can be learned in that way. Furthermore, there is good evidence that people in clinical trials do better than people not in clinical trials, probably for these reasons: clinical trials are usually done by the best experts in the field; individuals in clinical trials get more testing and closer follow-up and attention; and individuals in clinical trials know they are being closely watched and are more likely to do the things that are good for them, such as following their diet, quitting smoking, and taking their medications.

Part 2
What You Can Do

6

Risk Factors, Old and New

Traditional Risk Factors

Heart attacks and strokes in North America have declined by 60 percent (after adjusting for age) since early in the twentieth century. For the most part, this improvement has been due to a reduction in the traditional risk factors. These risk factors were identified in the Framingham Heart Study, in which the population of Framingham, Massachusetts, just west of Boston, has been followed for more than fifty years, with regular research examinations. In that study it became apparent that independent predictors of risk included age, being male, smoking, high blood pressure, thickening of the heart muscle (left ventricular hypertrophy), high blood cholesterol, and glucose intolerance (diabetes and prediabetes).

These risk factors interact strongly. Having more than one increases the risk in a way that is more than additive; the risk factors multiply each other. They also interact differently at different ages, and somewhat differently in men than in women. Not only is the risk of a heart attack much higher in men and women over age sixty-five, even those with low blood pressure, but also the relative risk rises much more steeply in older people as blood pressure increases. Furthermore, the prevalence of high blood pressure increases remarkably with age: whereas about 30 percent of people in the general population have high blood pressure, about 60 percent of people age eighty and above have at least isolated systolic high blood pressure—systolic pressure above 160 with diastolic pressure less than 90 mmHg. (The systolic pressure, the higher and first number in a blood pressure reading, measures the force that blood exerts on the artery walls as the heart contracts to pump out the blood. The diastolic pressure, the lower and second number in a reading, measures the force during relaxation of the heart.)

Since we can't change our age or sex, we need to work on the other risk factors. Among these, the most important is smoking. Smoking increases the risk of stroke six-fold; even living or working with smokers nearly doubles the risk. The reasons that smoke is so harmful are not all known; as there are several thousand chemicals in smoke, the problem is complex.

Smoking

Tobacco smoke is an incredibly complicated mix of some three thousand poisons, including benzene, ammonia, nicotine, tars, and carbon monoxide.

Probably very few of us are not exposed to tobacco smoke at all. Living with a smoker, or working in an environment with smokers, exposes us to a risk equal to smoking nearly half a pack of cigarettes ourselves, so it is not a simple matter to identify a true nonsmoker. In part, this is probably why it was difficult for researchers to show that spouses of smokers are at increased risk: there is so much background exposure in the workplace and in other public places that it was tricky to separate that from exposure at home.

The children of smokers are also at increased risk: babies born to smoking mothers show the earliest lesions of atherosclerosis in their umbilical arteries; they are also much more likely to have retarded growth in the uterus and to be born prematurely, and to suffer the risks associated with these problems. Compared to children of nonsmokers, children of smokers are more likely to suffer crib death and three times more likely to have serious lung problems, including asthma and infections; by age fourteen, boys who live with smoking parents already have enlarged hearts.

Which of the many toxins in tobacco smoke are responsible for vascular disease is not entirely known, but carbon monoxide is a strong candidate. Carbon monoxide is an odorless, colorless gas that you are familiar with as the toxic component of automobile exhaust fumes. It binds to the hemoglobin in your red blood cells two hundred times as firmly as oxygen does, and it thus displaces oxygen from your bloodstream.

Just being in a room with smokers for two hours raises your blood level of carbon monoxide to the equivalent of twice the safety level allowed in industry. At that point, the oxygen level in your blood is about what it would be on the top of a mile-high mountain. Carbon monoxide binds so firmly to the hemoglobin that it takes about sixteen hours to be eliminated; anyone exposed to tobacco smoke for a good part of each day, therefore, always has an abnormally high level of carbon monoxide in the blood.

SMOKING AND CORONARY ARTERY DISEASE

Because the oxygen-carrying capacity of the blood is reduced by carbon monoxide, exposure even to the smoke of others is especially harmful for individuals with coronary artery disease. Patients who have angina pectoris (chest pain brought on by exertion, due to narrowing of the coronary arteries) have a reduced capacity to exercise when exposed to the smoke of others, as a study by Dr. Wilbert Aronow and colleagues in the United States showed: persons with angina exposed to tobacco smoke in a poorly ventilated room had a 38 percent reduction in their ability to exercise, and those exposed to the smoke of others even in a well-ventilated room had a 22 percent reduction in the length of time that they could exercise on a treadmill before they developed chest pain.

Whatever it is in tobacco smoke that causes disease of the blood vessels, individuals who smoke develop artery blockage significantly faster, and have a significantly increased risk of having a heart attack or stroke, than do nonsmokers. Men who smoke have less than half the chance of nonsmokers to collect a nickel of their pensions.

It is clear that if you quit smoking, you reduce your risk of heart attack by half, and the benefit occurs within months. (It takes longer, perhaps ten years, to reduce the risk of developing cancer from smoking.)

High Blood Pressure (Hypertension)

One of the biggest advances in prevention has been the revolution in detecting and treating high blood pressure. *Hypertension* means simply "high blood pressure"; it does not imply nervousness or stress, although stress probably does aggravate high blood pressure.

Blood pressure is usually measured by inflating a cuff that is connected to a column of mercury, or to a mechanical device that simulates a column of mercury. A stethoscope is placed over the brachial artery at the elbow; the cuff is wrapped around the upper arm and inflated until the artery is compressed so firmly that blood can't get through, and then the cuff is deflated. Listening through the stethoscope over the artery reveals a tapping sound when the pressure of the blood in the artery is enough to push blood through, and the tapping sound goes away when the artery stays open between beats. Because the pressure wave is generated by the contraction of the heart (systole), the top pressure is called systolic pressure; when the artery stays open between beats, which corresponds to the relaxation phase of the heart (diastole), this is called diastolic pressure.

Both readings are important; it is a great myth that the diastolic pressure matters more. In fact, because the elderly are at higher risk, treating isolated systolic pressure in the elderly achieves more reduction in risk over a few years than does treating moderate diastolic pressure in younger people.

High blood pressure is aggravated by high salt intake, by obesity, and by ingesting certain substances such as alcohol, licorice, decongestants, birth-control pills, and arthritis pills. Stress also aggravates high blood pressure, but the interaction is complicated. In the short term, blood pressure goes up and back down again after exposure to an acute stress, such as an explosion.

It is commonly believed that long-term stress does not cause hypertension, but I have seen too many cases of medium-term (up to a year) worsening of blood pressure related to stress to regard it as a minor problem. The first time I observed this was in a young man who on his first visit to the clinic had a pressure of 240/140. (An ideal blood pressure would be below 120/80.) He was admitted to a hospital right away, where his wife's lawyer served him with divorce papers that afternoon. For three years his blood pressure was very hard to control, partly because his asthma limited the choice of medication that he could take. His pressure was seldom better than 180/100, despite his taking about seven blood-pressure pills per day. Three years later he came into the clinic with a pressure of 120/80, having reduced his pills to a half tablet a day of a diuretic (water pill). When I asked him what had changed, he replied that he and his wife had been back together for several months. He had never gotten closure on their separation, and the stress kept his pressure up until his personal situation resolved.

In other individuals, I have seen divorce, death of a spouse, loss of a job, loss of a house, and other major life events aggravate hypertension for months and even years. In such situations it is likely that receiving grief counseling, sharing feelings with friends or family members, or receiving professional stress-management counseling may help. There is evidence that stress management can lower blood pressure, at least in the medium term.

Cholesterol and Lipids

The word *cholesterol* is often used as shorthand for the profile of fats in the blood, including cholesterol, triglycerides, saturated fats, trans-fatty acids, and other harmful substances from food. In fact, cholesterol is not a fat; it is a steroid molecule produced by the body and ingested only in meat. One collective name for fats is *lipids*.

Because fat is not soluble in water, and blood is mostly water, we need a way to transport fats in the blood. Fat from food goes from the intestine to the liver in lymphatic fluid, and is then taken out of the blood by cells in the liver. It travels in the bloodstream in packages made up of an outer layer of protein, with fat in the center. These proteins are called *lipoproteins* (proteins that transport lipids), and vascular risk has as much to do with the lipoproteins as it does with the lipids themselves.

Because the lipoproteins are hard to measure, we are still learning about them; what is measured in routine lab testing is actually a combination of lipids alone and the lipids contained in lipoproteins. A common lipid profile consists of measurement of levels of total cholesterol, triglycerides, and high-density lipoprotein cholesterol (HDL—"good"—cholesterol). From this profile the level of low-density lipoprotein cholesterol (LDL—"bad"—cholesterol) is usually calculated. It is important to know that if triglycerides are above a certain level, the calculated LDL is invalid.

Estimation of risk is very tricky, and much more complicated than most people (including most doctors) think. In general, it is safe to say that the level of LDL is a better way to predict risk than the total cholesterol level; the ratio of total cholesterol to HDL is even more telling. A high level of Apolipoprotein A may be a stronger predictor still, but this is rarely measured. High triglycerides are an independent predictor of risk, but this measure is complicated by the fact that if triglycerides are high, HDL is usually low. A particularly high-risk profile is a high triglyceride level with low HDL and high LDL cholesterol. That profile often is associated with diabetes, or a state that precedes diabetes called *insulin resistance.*

Diabetes Mellitus

In Greek, *diabetes* means "excess urination," and *mellitus* (from honey) means "sweet"; thus diabetes mellitus got its name in ancient times from Greek physicians who noted that the urine of affected individuals tasted sweet, because there was sugar in the urine. Here we will simply use the term *diabetes.* (There are causes of diabetes besides a high level of sugar in the blood, including *diabetes insipidus*—the urine tasted insipid to the Greek physicians because it was dilute; a pituitary gland problem is the usual cause.)

Obesity is increasing rapidly in North America, and diabetes is expected to double in the next ten years or so as a result. Diabetes is the commonest cause of blindness and kidney failure in our society. It is also a strong risk factor for heart attacks and strokes: diabetics who have not had a heart attack have as high a risk as people who have had one.

There are two kinds of diabetes mellitus. Insulin deficiency or juvenile diabetes is called Type I; insulin resistance, called Type II, is the kind that comes on with age and is much more common.

TYPE II DIABETES

In a healthy person, insulin (a hormone) from the pancreas causes sugar to enter cells throughout the body. Sugar is produced from dietary carbohydrates (starchy foods) and other sources of energy by metabolism in the liver. In type I diabetes, the pancreas is unable to produce insulin, and blood sugar levels rise. A simplified explanation of what brings on Type II diabetes is that the body becomes increasingly resistant to the effects of insulin; insulin levels have to go higher and higher to keep the blood sugar normal, and at some point the pancreas can't keep up and the blood sugar rises. Recently some individuals have been regarded as having both Type I and Type II diabetes; this has been called *double diabetes*.

The best treatment for Type II diabetes is weight loss and exercise. Here the purpose of the exercise is not only to help with weight loss but also, in a sense, to retrain the muscles to respond to a more normal insulin level.

There are three kinds of pills used to treat Type II diabetes: the glitazones (thiazolidinediones), such as pioglitazone and rosiglitazone, which help restore the body's sensitivity to insulin; metformin, which reduces the amount of sugar produced by the liver; and the sulphonylureas, such as glyburide, which increase the amount of insulin released by the pancreas. These drugs are more effective when used in combination.

Sometimes insulin by injection or nasal spray may be needed for Type II diabetes because the blood-sugar levels can't be controlled without it, but this treatment leads to a vicious circle: the insulin makes people hungry, so it is harder to lose weight. Insulin treatment also aggravates insulin resistance. For those reasons weight loss and exercise are in principle the better treatment, and it is really worth doing them effectively.

New Risk Factors

The traditional risk factors explain only half of the incidence of blockage in the carotid arteries (atherosclerosis), and about half of the risk of heart attacks.

Genetic factors also contribute to risk. Heart attacks and strokes run in families; Swedish twin studies showed that about 80 percent of the risk of heart attacks was inherited. Some of this risk is due to inheritance of such factors as high cholesterol levels and high blood pressure, but much (about half) is due to genetic factors not yet known. With the completion of the Human Genome Project, in which the sequence of the entire human genome has been recorded, we have an incredible tool kit available to discover new causes of atherosclerosis, and thereby discover new treatments for it.

Some of the new risk factors that have been uncovered include a transport protein for lipids called lipoprotein (a) and an amino acid, homocysteine, that is elevated in people deficient in vitamin B_{12} and for many other reasons (discussed in a later chapter). Infections including Chlamydia pneumoniae are being investigated as factors that may contribute to vascular risk, and a marker of inflammation called C-reactive protein (CRP) appears to be associated with increased risk of heart attacks. Much has been made of CRP and the effect of cholesterol-lowering drugs on CRP, but in my view much of this is hype related to marketing. We have no specific treatment for CRP, including cholesterol-lowering drugs, so I do not see much benefit in measuring it. (Measuring CRP identifies high-risk people, but as described in an earlier chapter, measuring the plaque in the arteries is a much better indicator.)

Equally interesting are inherited factors that protect a person from atherosclerosis. The first was discovered by Cesare Sirtori and his colleagues in Milan, who discovered in a small hill town in Italy (isolated because there was no road in to the town until the 1950s) a large, long-lived family with very low levels of "good" cholesterol (high-density lipoprotein or HDL cholesterol). Studies of the family uncovered a mutation called the ApoA1Milano dimer, which was protective. In essence, the HDL in this family is super-effective, so even low levels are protective. When an artificial form of the super-HDL was given intravenously to people with coronary disease, it regressed the coronary plaque within weeks; news reports called it Drano for the arteries. Research is ongoing into how to make such treatment practical. Another recently discovered protective factor related to cholesterol was found to be more common in African Americans.

In my lab we have begun searching for new risk factors, and the treatments they will lead to, by using plaque measurement to quantify the extent to which individuals have excess atherosclerosis not explained by traditional risk factors ("unexplained atherosclerosis"), or who enjoy protection from atherosclerosis. We have used this approach to study a number of genes suspected of contributing to excess atherosclerosis; the real payoff will come from studies called *linkage studies* to identify previously unsuspected genetic causes of atherosclerosis and treatments for them.

Quitting Smoking

Claims that illness from tobacco smoke is the number-one preventable health problem in our society may surprise us. The basis of such claims, however, is that tobacco smoke is not only one of the main risk factors for heart attack and stroke but also one of the few that we can do something about, and the only one that can be entirely cured.

Quitting smoking reduces your risk of heart attack and stroke by *half* within six months. It is more effective, more quickly, than any medical treatment available. (Dietary change reduces strokes by about half, but it takes about four years; medications to lower cholesterol can reduce risk of stroke by about 30 percent in four years; and treating high blood pressure will reduce stroke by 40–50 percent in four years.)   What all this means is that if you have hardening of the arteries, or if you have other risk factors such as a family history of artery disease, high blood pressure, or high cholesterol, *quitting smoking is the most important health measure you can take.* For some reason, high levels of the amino acid homocysteine interact particularly strongly with smoking. If you already have other risk factors and artery disease, you simply can't afford to keep smoking. You need to decide that you *must* quit.

The secret is that there is a big difference between quitting and trying to quit. Trying to quit goes on forever. You tell your friends who offer you a cigarette, "No thanks, I'm trying to quit." You then take a cigarette, and after you take a few from a number of friends, you have to buy a pack to pay them all back, and so it goes. Quitting smoking is different from trying to quit. The basis for making it happen is to stop thinking of it as trying to quit, and make up your mind that you will quit.

What you need to embrace is the parable of the cold lake: if you are walking along the shore of a cold lake and see one of your grandchildren drowning, it takes no will power to go into the lake. It just has to be done. If you have vascular disease, you need to think of quitting smoking as something that *has* to be done—*it doesn't take will power to do something that must be done.*

The question is how to do it. The answer differs by individual. Some people are group oriented and will benefit from participating in smoke-ending groups or Y-Smoke groups at the YM/YWCA. Others are private individuals who would be better quitting on their own. Some people can quit only cold turkey, whereas for others quitting cold turkey is too difficult.

For those who have great difficulty quitting because of addiction to nicotine, the use of nicotine patches together with a medication such as bupropion (Zyban) may be optimal while quitting cold turkey. Other more effective medications are in development. If you choose that method, you should understand that while you are wearing the nicotine patch, you should stop smoking completely. It is important, though, not to think of the patch and bupropion as the magic switch for quitting: the magic switch is making up your mind not to take the first one, no matter how hard it is. Once you do that, the hard part will be over in three weeks.

For others, particularly those who cannot stop completely while wearing a patch, a program of gradual smoking cessation with behavior modification and a nicotine substitute such as nicotine gum is more effective, as described next.

Why Is It So Hard to Quit?

Smoking is a complex behavior. It is not only a physical addiction to nicotine but also a social activity. How often have you been in a room with a number of people, of whom a few are smokers, and seen that when one smoker lights up, the others all light up together? There is a social aspect to smoking, and if you smoke, there are certain situations that you associate with smoking. Many people have difficulty not smoking if they have coffee or an alcoholic drink, or if they are playing cards with friends. One patient of mine who had an especially hard time quitting smoking worked at a cookie factory, where all her co-workers smoked. Lighting up together was an important social aspect of their work breaks; when she quit smoking, she was ostracized during the breaks.

How Can You Quit?

The key to quitting is to make up your mind that you *must* and *will* quit. Recognize that if you smoke a pack or more of cigarettes a day, you are not really smoking them, but lighting them and burning them in ashtrays. Often, a cigarette gets lit by magic when the telephone rings—you find yourself talking on the phone with a cigarette in your hand wondering how it got lit. These magically lit cigarettes are the easiest to eliminate, since they are lit by habit, and mainly not smoked but burned in ashtrays.

It will be surprisingly easy to go from a pack a day to around five cigarettes a day if you can have something to help the craving in between those scheduled cigarettes. Get some nicotine patches and/or gum. Begin your schedule with five cigarettes a day, and actually write down the times that you will allow yourself a cigarette during the first week. For example, write on your calendar on one day of the week, such as Sunday, that you are going to smoke five cigarettes per day for the next week, and the times you will smoke them. Smoke these five cigarettes when it is time, whether you want them or not, and in between those times, no matter how much you want a cigarette, chew the nicotine gum instead.

If you have trouble with a sore mouth or nausea from the nicotine gum, it will help to chew it more slowly; use it more like a lozenge, with an occasional bite on the gum to get a squirt of nicotine, or use nicotine patches or nasal spray instead.

Each week eliminate one cigarette, so you get down to four a day the second week, three a day the third week, and zero after five weeks. Mark the day you will quit on the calendar in advance, and plan a celebration to mark the day when you do the most important thing for your health that you can do.

Expect that this will begin a difficult time for you and that you will actually experience a period of mourning. Plan to minimize that mourning experience by combating it with a celebration. Invite some friends over, or go out for dinner and spend some of the money you will save by not smoking. Commit yourself to quitting by telling your friends that you are quitting, and ask them to help you in this important change rather than to make it difficult for you. Then make up your mind that you have quit smoking, and never take another cigarette. If you never take the first one, you won't start again.

The most difficult time may be the first two or three weeks after you quit. You may become irritable and moody, and your family and friends may say something like, "For heaven's sake, you're too hard to live with, why don't you start smoking again?" During that time, it may be reasonable for you to request from your physician a prescription for a mild tranquilizer or for bupropion (Zyban), an antidepressant. If the alternative is to go back to smoking, it is much healthier for you to use a tranquilizer for a couple of weeks. Be careful, however, to avoid combining tranquilizers with alcohol, particularly when you have to drive, operate heavy machinery, or be in other hazardous situations.

It may also be helpful to work with a psychologist or a smoking-cessation program for help with understanding why you smoke, why it is so difficult to quit, and how you can deal with the stress of quitting.

Are Nicotine Substitutes Harmful?

You may be concerned about whether nicotine gum or other substitutes such as patches are harmful. Most people get about two to four milligrams of nicotine from a cigarette (depending on how often and how deeply they take a draw); therefore a piece of nicotine gum with two to four milligrams of nicotine has about the same amount of nicotine as a cigarette, and a high-dose (twenty-one milligrams) nicotine patch is about the same as a half pack of cigarettes. The nicotine substitute, however, does not have the carbon monoxide, or the three thousand or so other poisons contained in cigarette smoke. If the alternative to a nicotine substitute is a cigarette, the gum or patch is much safer.

Losing Weight

Weight loss has been politicized in the last few years, so I need to begin by saying that for people at risk of strokes, weight control is a health issue. I am not talking here about trying to look like a magazine centerfold, I am talking about preventing strokes! I should probably also mention my credentials: I am one of those former football players who got fat when I quit playing. I have kept fifty pounds off for forty years (since the end of my internship, when I had ballooned up from drinking a lot of coffee with sugar in it and eating doughnuts to keep myself awake on long shifts). I am therefore one of those people who gain a pound walking past a bakery; I know how hard losing weight is, and I know what works.

How to Lose Weight and Keep It Off

Dieting is not the answer to weight control; in fact there is evidence that cyclic dieting may aggravate obesity. The only realistic way to lose weight and keep it off is to permanently reduce calorie intake below energy consumption. Thus, the key to success in this difficult arena is to stop thinking in terms of a temporary change in eating patterns—a "diet"—and to permanently change your approach to meal planning. If the foods you grew up with are too much for your body to handle, it follows that you need to learn a different pattern of eating; the trick is learning how to make healthy food enjoyable, rather than thinking in negative terms (such as, "Now I have to cut out everything I like").

ENERGY IN, ENERGY OUT

The basis of weight control is the first law of thermodynamics: energy can neither be created nor destroyed. What determines your weight is the balance between energy intake and energy consumption. If you eat more calories than you burn off, you will gain weight, and if you burn off more calories than you eat, you will lose weight.

Sorry, there is no magic. There is no such thing as putting weight on without eating more calories than are expended. The difficulty may be in part that some of us are born with more efficient bodies and do not seem to burn as many calories as others. A recent theory is that obesity in some people may be due to abnormal fat metabolism resulting from a genetic defect in the beta-3 type of receptors to adrenaline. In others, it may be related to abnormalities in leptin, or leptin receptors, or ghrelin. Whatever the cause, we who have the problem have only one solution: to lose weight we need either to eat fewer calories than others, or to burn more calories than others.

People often say that they are overweight because they don't exercise as much as they used to. They point to a sprained ankle, a new job, or some other reason to explain their weight gain. There is seldom as much truth in this as people think. To burn off the hundred calories in four crackers, you have to run a six-minute mile; it's a lot easier to skip the crackers. To burn off a significant number of calories on a weekly basis requires an unusual amount of athletic activity. Marathon runners, stevedores, and lumberjacks burn enough energy to allow them to eat more than sedentary city dwellers do, but most people with a sedentary occupation, even if they have a routine of exercise several times a week, need to control their weight by also controlling their calorie intake.

NO DIETING

The fundamental basis of weight control, therefore, is to *permanently* restrict calorie intake. This is different from a diet, if you think of diet as a temporary change in eating habits.

One pound of fat contains 3,500 calories. This means that to lose one pound of fat you need to cut out 500 calories a day for seven days from your normal calorie intake. To lose fifty pounds, you need to cut 500 calories a day for fifty weeks (i.e., a year); to keep it off, you need to cut out 500 calories per day permanently. The average sedentary person burns about 10 calories per pound every day; this means that 2,000 calories per day sustains a weight of about 200 pounds. It is pretty likely that people who have trouble with overweight burn fewer calories than does the average person. This means that to maintain a healthy weight, we need to permanently eat fewer calories. The key to making this work is to eat more low-calorie foods and fewer high-calorie foods. To do this, we need to know the calorie values of the foods we eat.

The Price-Tag Approach

Learn to think of your daily calorie intake as an allowance of hard-earned money. Set your allowance at the number of calories per day that you need to lose a pound a week, and stick to that many calories per day. For instance, if you wake up every morning with 1,500 calories to spend, it helps to think of the calorie counts of the foods that you may consider eating as the price tag. If someone says, "Let's go to McDonald's and have a Big Mac and fries," you have to know that will cost you more than 1,000 calories. If you have already eaten 300 calories for breakfast and plan to consume 700 calories for dinner, you cannot afford to blow 1,000 calories on lunch.

Most people eat when they want to, and they eat what they want to. This is the way to caloric bankruptcy; it is like going to Wal-Mart with a credit card and buying anything you like without regard to the cost. To stay on a calorie budget, you have to look at the price tag. It helps to think in terms of not wasting your calories on things you don't really want. Save those hard-earned calories for something really enjoyable.

This does not mean that you can never have cake and ice cream, but it means that if you want to have cake and ice cream, you have to budget for it. When you realize that a wedge of cake and two scoops of ice cream will cost you 800 calories, you will understand that you cannot have cake and ice cream for dessert—you will have to have them for dinner, with some calories saved up from lunch!

Calorie Bombs

Many foods have surprisingly high calorie counts, and one trick to keeping weight off is to know what they are. I call them calorie bombs. Reduce your intake of high-calorie foods and find some low-calorie foods that you can enjoy, so that you won't feel starved and deprived. "A Guide to Healthy Meals" at the end of this book includes recipes and cooking techniques for learning how to make tasty and interesting vegetable dishes. The reason for this is that meat is very fattening, and our society tends to base meals on meat.

My "calorie clock" divides foods into four groups according to their calorie counts (Figure 6.1):

1. Green vegetables such as spinach, lettuce, broccoli, celery, etc., with zero calories
2. Vegetables with a bit of sugar such as carrots and peas (corn is more like a starch), with 50 calories per half-cup, an average serving
3. Starches and sugars, such as potatoes, pasta, rice, and the "optional" sugars and starches (not part of the main meal) such as bread, juice, fruit, four crackers, or half a bagel, which are each 100 calories per average serving

4. Foods with fat in them, such as meat, cake, pie, ice cream, nuts, doughnuts, large muffins, and fried foods such as potato chips or French fries, which are around 400 calories per average serving

To lose weight and keep it off, you need to eat a lot more of the no-calorie and 50-calorie foods, eat a lot less of the 400-calorie foods, and control the sugars and starches. If you keep to one starch with your main meal and five or six of the "optional" sugars and starches, keep your intake of animals to two ounces a day or four ounces every other day, and avoid the "calorie bombs" such as cake, pie, ice cream, chips, and fries, you will lose weight.

MEAT, NUTS, CHIPS, FRIES, AND SALAD DRESSING

A four-ounce serving of meat contains 300–400 calories, about the same as a chocolate bar. Nobody trying to lose weight would be foolish enough to start a meal by putting two chocolate bars on the plate, but how often have you heard someone say, "I'm trying to lose weight, so I'll skip the baked potato and have an extra pork chop instead"? Unfortunately, a medium/large baked potato is only 200 calories, whereas the pork chop is 350–400!

The reason for the difference is that fat and oil in meat have more than twice the calories of the carbohydrates in the potato, and meat has fat and cholesterol all through it, even if you trim off the visible fat. One gram of fat or oil contains 9 calories, whereas a gram of carbohydrates or protein has only 4 calories. Thus, foods that contain fat or oil are a problem. One peanut contains 7 calories, one cashew contains 15 calories, and a large olive has 35 calories. A teaspoon of oil is about 45 calories, so a tablespoon of salad dressing is about 120 calories. There are commercially available low-fat salad dressings, but if you have high blood pressure you need to watch their salt content. (See the recipe for low-calorie salad dressing in "A Guide to Healthy Meals" at the end of the book).

FRUIT, JUICE, AND BREAD

Another problem is sugar, which can be packed into foods in surprisingly large amounts because it dissolves in water. Cake and ice cream are fairly obvious, although ice cream has the added problem

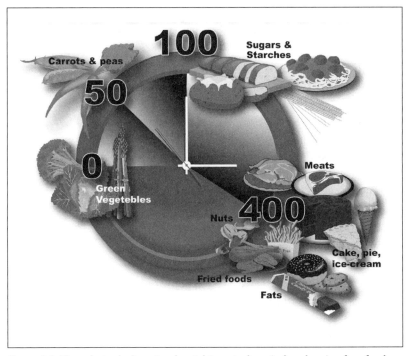

Figure 6.1 The calorie clock, a visual weight-control reminder, showing four food groups by calorie count

that it contains fat. Two scoops of ice cream will cost you about 400 calories! Less obvious is fruit, which has a fair amount of sugar in it. We tend to think of fruit as healthy, but one grape contains 4 calories (and so does one raisin), and a glass of orange juice (a kitchen tumbler, not a small juice glass) contains 100 calories, as does a glass of soda pop. Most average servings of fruit are about 100 calories.

A slice of bread is only about 100 calories, but each teaspoon of margarine is about 50 calories, a teaspoon of peanut butter is about 40 calories, and a level teaspoon of jam is about 25.

If you have a sweet tooth, you may need to buy fewer sweet things, because if they are in the house, you will eat them. Learn to use artificial sweetener such as sucralose (Splenda) to satisfy your sweet tooth. Use Jell-O made with sweetener as a dessert. Use sweetener in beverages such as coffee, and to make lemonade. You can even use sucralose in baking. In my view, sucralose is the best sugar substitute; it is actually a kind of sugar that we can't absorb, so it tastes more like sugar and cooks more like sugar.

FRIED FOODS

Oil sticks to foods when you fry them. A doughnut contains about 100 calories of flour and sugar, but once you drop it into a deep-fat fryer and pull it out again, it zooms to 250 calories. A large baked potato is 200 calories, but cut up as fries it soaks up 400 additional calories of bad fat. A single potato chip has such a huge surface area that although it contains only 1 calorie of potato, it soaks up 9 calories of fat!

Boiling, broiling, roasting, and microwaving are ways to cook food instead of frying.

When stir-frying, use the minimum amount of oil you can get by with. It helps to use a nonstick wok and to spray the cooking dish with a vegetable oil (like Pam) to prevent things from sticking. A 1.5-second spray is 7 calories, compared to 50 calories for a teaspoon of oil. Keep some water and a spoon handy to add a bit of water to the wok if food is sticking.

ALCOHOL

Not only is alcohol bad for blood pressure, bad for your liver, and capable of ruining your life if you drink too much of it or drink it at the wrong time, but also it is fattening. An ounce of liquor contains about 100 calories, a beer about 150, and a glass of wine between 100 and 200, depending on the size. A mixed drink such as an ounce and a half of rum and ten ounces of cola will cost you about 250 calories, as will the refill. If losing a pound a week requires cutting out only 500 calories a day, you may only need to cut out two mixed drinks or three beers a day!

What's Left?

How do you keep from starving if you cut down your meat intake to one two-ounce serving a day (or four ounces every other day)? The plan is basically to eat more low-calorie foods, and fewer high-calorie foods. This means eating mainly vegetables, and only a little bit of meat, bread, and fruit. In flavoring foods, you need to find low-calorie alternatives that you can enjoy. For example, instead of topping a baked potato with the butter and sour cream that add several hundred calories, use a small bit of canola margarine and, if you enjoy sour cream, a bit of non-fat sour cream, or low-fat yogurt, or buttermilk. (Buttermilk is equivalent in fat and calories to skim milk). Vegetables are mainly cellulose and water, so they are very low in calories as long as you don't smother them with butter or cheese sauce. Learn to make tasty and interesting dishes in a wok (see "A Guide to Healthy Meals") or microwave; try frozen vegetables for convenient variety. Use popcorn instead of potato chips or nuts, and switch to half a bagel instead of a doughnut.

The Bottom Line

Do not think of a weight-reduction program as a punishment, or as a temporary change in eating habits. If you are overweight, you need to make a *permanent* lifetime modification in the way you think about food. To lose a pound a week requires cutting out about 500 calories a day from your previous intake. You need to reduce your intake of high-calorie foods, but you are unlikely to stick with this unless you find low-calorie substitutes that you can enjoy. "A Guide to Healthy Meals" offers ideas for how to make low-fat choices enjoyable. It is much easier to reduce your calorie intake than to burn off more calories, but an exercise program helps in other ways, as we see next.

Exercise

It is easy to either overestimate or underestimate the benefits of exercise. Often, people who decide to take up exercise for health reasons go at it too hard at first, have an injury such as a pulled tendon, and quit. Until recently, there was more enthusiasm and fad than solid knowledge involved in the promotion of exercise; a lot of misinformation and confusion still exists.

The Benefits

Exercise should be considered part of the nondrug management of blood pressure, diabetes, and cholesterol. There is some evidence now that exercise programs do improve survival among people who have had a heart attack; this probably also applies to people who have had a stroke.

One of the first studies to suggest the benefits of exercise was the London bus drivers' study about thirty-five years ago. The investigators compared the drivers and conductors on the big red double-decker buses in London, England. They found that, in comparison to bus conductors, drivers had more heart attacks and died younger; they concluded that the reason was probably that the driver sat behind the wheel all day, while the conductor ran up and down the stairs taking tickets. (It's possible that there were other reasons: our research on stress, discussed later in this chapter, suggests that if the driver was experiencing a lot more stress, which is pretty likely, the excess of vascular events may not have been due entirely to the difference in exercise.) Several other retrospective studies have suggested that exercise is beneficial, but it is hard to control for all the other behaviors (diet, smoking) and other factors such as education that affect risk, and to be sure that exercise is the main reason for the differences observed.

There is good evidence that exercise, in addition to enhancing well-being and quality of life, improves a number of the risk factors for heart attack and stroke: blood pressure, diabetes, and the level of HDL in the blood. Some evidence also exists, from controlled trials, of improved outcomes with exercise among people who have survived a heart attack.

How Much, How Often, and What Kind?

There is a point of diminishing returns with exercise. More may be better, but a lot of exercise isn't all that much better than a moderate amount. You get most of the benefit of exercise from the equivalent of a half hour a day of brisk walking, or a moderately hard forty-five-minute workout three times a week. Brisk walking means a pace of two miles (about three kilometers) per half-hour.

The type of exercise is important. Aerobic exercise is better than power lifting, which in fact may aggravate blood pressure. If you want to work out at a gym on Nautilus-type machines, plan to keep the weights low enough that you can do about thirty repeats, or even more with some of the large muscle groups such as abdominal muscles. Don't do weights or machines on consecutive days; take a rest day in between. A good program includes an aerobic workout (a brisk walk, stair climber, treadmill, exercise bike, swimming, or aerobics class) and on alternate days a workout on machines such as Nautilus equipment. Try to work out a few days a week, with a minimum of a moderate forty-five-minute aerobic workout three days a week, or a half-hour brisk walk daily.

If you hate exercise, look for ways to make it fun or do something else at the same time, such as watching TV. If you can get into an active sport such as squash or tennis and have fun at the same time, so much the better. Don't kid yourself, though, that games such as bowling will do much for you. Golf is a special case. If you ride a cart and play on a course where play is very slow, there won't be much benefit; if you walk briskly and push or carry your own bag, there is a reasonable workout in a round—especially if your game isn't very accurate and you go back and forth across the fairway. The average course is about six thousand yards, about a four-mile walk. (I find that at the end of summer when I go back to the gym after a season of golf, I can still do about 80 percent of my peak spring fitness level on a stair climber, which is pretty good.)

A very important principle is to start off with something easy and work up very gradually: don't overdo it, pull a tendon, and end up quitting. Never increase both the intensity and duration of exercise at the same time. If you are doing a certain level on something like a stair climber, do the same workout for a week before increasing either the duration or intensity, and make the increments small. For example, if you start off with ten minutes at level 6, increase your time by a minute a week until you are up to about twenty or twenty-five minutes, then try increasing the effort level by one grade every two weeks or so. If you are walking in your neighborhood, measure out a two-mile track. See how long it takes you to walk two miles at a comfortable pace, and then try to take off a minute a week until you can walk two miles in a half hour; once you can do that comfortably, try going a bit farther each week.

You will find that getting in shape gives you more energy and general well-being; even if you aren't very enthusiastic at first, you will get to a place where you miss your exercise if you have to stop for some reason. Once that happens, you will be well on your way.

If you have trouble getting started, go to a fitness club or something like a YMCA; the fitness instructors at such places are usually very knowledgeable and will be able to help you plan a good program. If you are at risk of a heart attack, you may need to have a stress test done before embarking on an exercise program, to be sure that it's safe.

Managing Stress

It seems intuitively obvious that stress causes heart attacks and strokes—the terms *broken heart* and *apoplexy* (from the Greek *plēssein*, "to strike") reflect that folk belief.

Until recently, there has been little evidence to support that intuition. Robert Karasek (now in Lowell, Massachusetts) and Tom Pickering in New York have produced some evidence that lack of control over job demands and high time pressure on the job aggravate blood pressure. A fair amount of evidence links hostile Type A personality (highly time-driven, hostile people) to coronary risk, and Stephen Manuck in Pittsburgh and others have shown that people who have a marked rise in blood pressure during mental stress are at increased risk. There is also some evidence that mental stress induces changes on an electrocardiogram, indicating reduced blood flow to the heart muscle.

In 1997, Peter Barnett and I, with Steve Manuck and Richard Jennings from Pittsburgh, showed that the rise in blood pressure during mental stress induced by a frustrating computer game is a strong predictor of progression of carotid atherosclerosis (18). We had a group of 350 people with a wide range of atherosclerosis, ages twenty-eight to seventy-eight, play a computer game called the Stroop task. The task is frustrating and causes a marked rise in blood pressure in some people but not in others. We found that the rise in blood pressure during mental stress was a strong predictor of the rate of progression (worsening) of atherosclerotic plaque in the carotid arteries over two years.

A panel of the Canadian Hypertension Society (which I chaired) reviewed the literature on stress management and found that a comprehensive individualized program of stress management can reduce blood pressure, with effects lasting a year or so. To date there are no good large randomized trials showing that stress management reduces the occurrence of heart attacks or strokes.

In the meantime, it is likely that reducing your stress levels will be good for your blood pressure and probably for your arteries, not to mention for your enjoyment of life.

7
How to Manage Cholesterol

Thanks to the Framingham Heart Study, it has been clear for about twenty-five years that high blood levels of total cholesterol and triglycerides, high levels of low-density lipoprotein (LDL, or "bad," cholesterol) and low levels of high-density lipoprotein (HDL, or "good," cholesterol) are associated with increased risk of coronary disease. But only since 1994 has it also been clear that treating cholesterol will reduce coronary risk.

There is every reason to believe that strokes due to blocked arteries (atherosclerosis) will also be reduced significantly by treating cholesterol, although some controversy still exists about the relationship between cholesterol and stroke, because before we had CT scanning available to clearly distinguish between infarctions (tissue death due to permanent loss of blood flow) and hemorrhages, statistics tended to confuse or lump together strokes due to high blood pressure and strokes due to blocked arteries. Since the early 1980s revolution in blood-pressure detection and treatment, however, we know that blocked arteries cause about 75–80 percent of strokes, as well as heart attacks. Furthermore, it is now clear from the Veteran's Administration trial on asymptomatic carotid surgery (19) that persons with narrowing of the carotid arteries (carotid stenosis) have a very high risk of heart attacks; this means that people with carotid artery disease need their cholesterol treated to reduce coronary risk, in any case, as we will see.

Cholesterol Explained

Cholesterol is a sterol ring structure that is an important part of the membrane surrounding every cell in your body (sterols are solid steroid alcohols in lipids). You could not live without it. Cholesterol comes from two sources: your liver manufactures it, and you absorb it from your diet. When blood levels of cholesterol become elevated above the normal range, it's time to consider the source.

Cholesterol will not mix with water, so the body wraps it in protein to carry it in the blood; these packages, as we have seen, are called lipoproteins (proteins that transport lipids). The low-density lipoproteins, or LDL, carry approximately 70 per cent of the total cholesterol circulating in the blood. High levels of LDL are directly related a higher risk for developing coronary heart disease. It appears likely now that the really harmful form is oxidized LDL, and this has led to interest in antioxidant vitamins such as vitamin E, vitamin C, and beta-carotene. (Antioxidants are substances that inhibit oxidation, reactions promoted by oxygen.) You can picture how antioxidant vitamins work if you think what happens when a slice of apple or banana is exposed to air. It turns brown because of oxidation, but you can prevent this with a covering of lemon juice, because the vitamin C in the lemon juice is an antioxidant.

High-density lipoproteins, HDL, are protein-rich particles; 50 percent of their mass is protein. These carry cholesterol out of the bloodstream (and probably out of the artery wall) to the liver for processing, thereby lowering the risk of atherosclerosis. Diet changes and increased exercise can raise the percentage of HDL in the blood.

Routine blood tests indicate total cholesterol levels as well as the level of triglycerides in the blood. Triglycerides are sometimes referred to as a storage form of fat, since these either enter the fat tissue or are used by muscle cells as energy. One's level of triglycerides may be affected by the total energy value of one's diet and by the content of that diet. A diet which is typically high in fats and sugar (including alcohol) may contribute to overweight and, in turn, to high triglycerides.

It is now clear that we can reduce our risk of heart attack and stroke by consuming a Mediterranean diet, even if it does not lower the fasting level of cholesterol—the level of cholesterol in the blood-stream after a twelve-hour fast—the way our cholesterol is usually measured.

The reasons that a healthy diet is helpful are complicated, a com-bination of reducing problem foods and increasing protective ones. That is, a low-fat diet involves not just eating less animal fat, fatty acids, and cholesterol, but at the same time eating more substances that are protective, such as olive oil, nonhydrogenated canola mar-garine, whole grains, fruits, and vegetables. Fruits and vegetables are beneficial in part because they contain antioxidants, such as lycopene in tomato sauce. Indeed, lycopene is now trumpeted on the labels of some ketchup bottles.

Fasting versus Nonfasting Lipids

Although we routinely measure the level of cholesterol after a fast, the levels of cholesterol, fatty acids, other fats, and perhaps free radicals after meals are probably more important. (Free radicals are chemically active compounds that, among other negative reactions, oxidize LDL cholesterol.) The reason for measuring fasting levels is not that they are more informative but that they are less variable. It would be quite tricky to interpret postmeal levels without knowing the precise composition of the meal, and the precise timing of the blood sample after the meal was eaten; in fact, the key would be the timing of stomach emptying, which is quite variable.

I believe this issue has led to a great misunderstanding about the importance of diet. In most cases a healthy diet does not do much to reduce the level of fasting cholesterol. This is discouraging and may lead one to wonder, if a diet change doesn't do much, why bother?, and to conclude that it is okay to eat one's usual diet and take a pill to lower the fasting cholesterol. This is a big mistake, because diet has a major impact on the fats in the blood after meals (postmeal lipids), which are highly significant.

We are wrong to assume that a lab report indicating that our fasting lipids are in the normal range means that the lipid profile is acceptable. What we call a normal level in North America is about double the normal levels in China. Furthermore, fasting lipids don't tell the whole story (20).

There is increasing evidence that levels of fat and oxidized fat after meals (postmeal, or postprandial, lipids) are as important or more important than fasting lipids; perhaps it is because we spend about eighteen hours of the day in the fed state, and only a few hours a day in a state that reflects fasting lipid levels.

Similarly, the focus on "red meat" is based on the effect of saturated fat on liver metabolism on next morning's fasting lipids, and ignores the fact that the cholesterol is in the cell membrane of every muscle cell. Chicken (with the skin off) and fish have less saturated fat than beef, but just as much cholesterol.

Cholesterol in Our Diet

Eggs and Meat

There is a lot of confusion about dietary cholesterol, and in particular about egg yolks. One egg yolk contains about 275 mg of cholesterol (or 225 for the modern low-cholesterol chickens). Most dieticians tell people who have had a heart attack that it is okay to eat up to three eggs a week, based largely on the theory that because the body makes more cholesterol than we consume, body-produced cholesterol should be the focus and dietary cholesterol is not important. However, there is more to it than just the fasting level of ordinary LDL cholesterol. A study by Levy and colleagues in 1996 (21) showed that egg yolks (two a day for three weeks) raised the fasting level of ordinary LDL by only about 11 percent, but raised the fasting level of oxidized LDL by 34 percent: oxidized LDL is the harmful form of cholesterol. Think what is happening for the six hours or so after we eat the eggs! In 1999 an article in the *Journal of the American Medical Association* (22) reported that in high-risk people such as diabetics, an egg a day doubled coronary risk compared to less than one egg a week.

For people with bad arteries, target cholesterol intake should be around 100–125 mg/day (as in the Indo-Mediterranean diet study), so egg yolks, with 225–75 each, are out. The new eggs with omega-3 fatty acids get omega-3 into the eggs by feeding flaxseed to chickens.

However, they have almost as much cholesterol as regular eggs, so the answer is to eat the flaxseed yourself and leave the chicken out of it. Try egg substitutes made from egg whites, such as Egg Beaters or Better than Eggs, and so on. Sunday breakfast does not have to be boring just because it doesn't include egg yolks; some tasty recipes for omelets and frittata are included in "A Guide to Healthy Meals" at the end of the book.

Chinese who live in China have one-tenth the coronary risk North Americans have. They not only have fasting lipid levels that are half those of North Americans but also have a much smaller after-meal rise in fats and oxidative stress (free radicals that are chemically active and harm the function of the artery lining), as they eat mainly rice and vegetables. Chinese who live in North America have the same coronary risk as that of other North Americans. The reason is almost certainly that in China, where the average wage is about fifty dollars a month, people cannot afford much meat.

The Dean Ornish regression diet, which is extremely low in fat and includes little meat, has been shown to reduce the risk of coronary disease without drugs. The problem is that it is very hard for North Americans to stay on the diet, because we tend to name the meal by the meat. The question "What's for dinner tonight?" usually gets the answer "Chicken," or "Pork chops," or "Fish." We think of a meal as tasty meat with boring vegetables (such as peas, carrots, and potatoes with the flavor boiled out of them). If we try to reduce our intake of animal flesh to a pound a week, we can't conceive of only two ounces of meat on the plate along with boring vegetables.

Soluble Fiber

Your body makes more cholesterol every day than you would ever eat. As we have said, much of this is in the form of bile salts, which are stored in the gallbladder until mealtime. As soon as the food leaves the stomach and goes into the duodenum, a reflex contraction of the gallbladder pours the bile salts down the bile duct into the duodenum; they mix with the food and help with fat absorption as the food moves down the intestine. In the lower small bowel, the bile salts are reabsorbed, go back to the liver, and are stored in the bile duct. (If the gallbladder has been removed, the bile salts trickle into the intestine continuously.)

If your meal contains something that binds the bile salts and prevents them from being reabsorbed, the bile salts are eliminated in the stool, and your liver has to take cholesterol out of the bloodstream to make new bile salts.

Foods that are high in soluble fiber include oat bran (not wheat bran or All-bran—specifically oat bran), lentils, beans, broccoli, Brussels sprouts, okra, carrots, barley, and kiwi fruit. A good backup fiber, if you don't get one of the other sources in your meal, is psyllium powder or granules; one teaspoon of psyllium is equivalent to two to three tablespoons of oat bran. Try to include one of these options with each meal, and the effect will be to lower cholesterol by about 10 percent; that effect is big enough to reduce risk of heart attack (or strokes due to atherosclerosis) by about 20 percent.

The principle here is called *bile-acid sequestration* (that is, removal); resin powders (colestipol and cholestyramine) available as drugs work the same way, and ezetimibe also blocks the absorption of cholesterol by a different mechanism. (It specifically blocks cholesterol receptors in the lining of the intestine that are responsible for absorption of cholesterol.)

The Cretan Mediterranean Diet

The misplaced focus on fasting cholesterol, rather than on preventing heart attacks and strokes, has led most experts to recommend a low-fat diet because it reduces fasting cholesterol levels. The low-fat diet recommended currently in most coronary care units is the American Heart Association (AHA) diet—formerly the National Cholesterol Education Program, or NCEP, Step 2 diet—in which cholesterol intake is below 200 mg/day, and less than 20 percent of calories are from fat. This more restrictive diet is intended for patients who already have vascular disease. A more liberal (Step 1) diet, for people who do not yet have vascular disease, allows up to 300mg of cholesterol per day, and up to 30 percent of calories from fat. However, there is little or no evidence that this diet reduces heart attacks or strokes.

Three studies, however, have compared the AHA diet to a Mediterranean diet from the island of Crete. The first, in the early 1960s, was the Six Countries Study under the direction of Dr. Ancel Keys, which showed that on Crete people on average have their first heart attack at a much higher age than in other countries. Follow-up studies suggested that diet accounted for much of this improved survival. Two randomized controlled trials among survivors of heart attacks have since shown that a Cretan Mediterranean diet substantially reduces heart attacks, strokes, and deaths.

The second study, the Lyon Diet Heart Study, which compared a "prudent Western diet" similar to an NCEP Step 1 diet to a Cretan Mediterranean diet, showed that the Mediterranean diet reduced heart attacks and deaths by 60 percent in four years (23). More recently a study in India, the Indo-Mediterranean diet study, showed that a Mediterranean version of the Indian diet reduced heart attacks and strokes by half in two years, even though 60 percent of the participants were already vegetarians (24). The diet reduced the intake of animal flesh to about two ounces per day and of cholesterol to 125 mg/day, substituted soya oil and mustard oil for harmful oils in ghee (traditionally, clarified butter, now commonly replaced by hydrogenated vegetable oil), and increased the intake of fruits and vegetables. (Concerns about the legitimacy of this study have recently been answered.)

The Mediterranean Diet for North Americans

Eating only two ounces of animal flesh a day is a tall order for most North Americans. Most of my patients find it easier to go meatless every other day, and keep to four ounces total on the meat day: that means no tuna sandwich at noon if they are going to eat a piece of chicken at suppertime.

The trick is learning how to do it. You can use egg whites or substitutes such as Egg Beaters in virtually any recipe that calls for eggs. If you find plain Egg Beaters boring, chop in some green pepper and onion, and throw in a bit of mustard powder and Italian spice to make it tasty. And it's not enough to know a couple of tasty recipes, because they get boring pretty quickly; most households rotate about fifteen meals through the kitchen.

I encourage people to take a positive attitude, thinking of their meatless day every other day not as their punishment day but as their gourmet cooking-class day. You can learn how to make chili, pasta, stir-fries, barbecued vegetables, and other dishes without meat, and to make them delicious not with butter and cheese, but with herbs, spices, onions, green peppers, lemon juice, balsamic vinegar, and so on.

Very low-fat meals are a bit Spartan; we tend to miss the flavor of fat. A good trick is to use sesame oil, which has a strong nutty flavor—a few drops perk up a bowl of chili, a pasta dish, or grilled vegetables. Try a big portobello mushroom marinated in some Teriyaki sauce with a bit of balsamic vinegar, some mustard powder, fresh oregano, and a bit of sesame oil, and then barbecued—it's not that different from a steak.

The Bottom Line

The bottom line for individuals with atherosclerosis is a Cretan Mediterranean diet, which is high in olive oil and canola margarine, whole grains, fruits, vegetables, beans, lentils, chickpeas, and nuts, and low in cholesterol and animal fat (an animal, in this case, is anything with eyes, a face, or a mother; anything that walks, swims, flies, or crawls):

- Meat of any animal: two ounces per day or four ounces *every other day* (or less)
- *No* egg yolks; use egg substitutes
- Non-hydrogenated canola margarine and olive oil
- Whole-grain bread, cereals, and pasta; brown rice; fruits; vegetables
- Avoid fried foods: substitute bagels for doughnuts, popcorn for potato chips, a baked potato for french fries

Healthy Body Weight

What constitutes a healthy weight includes a wide range of possible weights based on appropriate eating habits, regular physical activity, and a realistic body weight. The Body Mass Index (BMI) has become a standard of reference for healthy adults between twenty and sixty-five years of age. BMI is calculated by dividing total weight in kilograms by height in meters squared (or by dividing weight in pounds by height in inches squared and multiplying the result by 703). It measures obesity to define health status.

For most people, a BMI of twenty to twenty-five is considered a healthy range. Those above or below this range may be at an increased risk for ill health. Maintaining lean weight is important because the larger your fat cells are, the more cholesterol your body makes.

Maintaining a healthy body weight is possible only by achieving a balance between energy (calorie) intake and energy output.

Designer Fuels for Our Bodies

If you and I were the zookeepers in the capital of Mars, and one of our spaceships returned from Earth after capturing a number of Earth creatures, we would have to not only provide housing for them but also figure out what they eat. If the ramp came down and out came elephants, giraffes, tigers, rabbits, and human beings, we would have to look at how their bodies differ in order to decide what they eat. The tigers, with fangs and claws, are obviously designed for eating meat; the camels and cows, with flat grinding teeth and ruminant stomachs, are designed for eating grass; the giraffes are designed for reaching up into trees to eat acacia leaves, and so on. If you think of how human beings are built (wimpy claws and fangs, flat grinding teeth like cows or camels, and a long intestine with a long appendix, like a rabbit's), it is clear that we are designed for eating mainly vegetables and occasionally a bit of meat. On a scale between rabbits and tigers, we are about two-thirds of the way toward rabbits. The problem is that our diet is about two-thirds of the way toward the tigers' diet. It's like running our engine on the wrong fuel: the valves get gummed up.

Our cave-dwelling ancestors who led a hunter-gatherer existence probably ate mainly leaves, berries, roots, fruit, and nuts; occasionally they chased an antelope for ten miles and if they got lucky they could eat it, but they burned off quite a lot in the chase.

I learned about healthy eating from two trips outside my usual world. The first was an expedition in the late 1970s to Northern Quebec near James Bay to study mercury poisoning among the Swampy Cree bands near Chibougamou. These aboriginal peoples live in reservations under the leadership of a band council, which controls the money from the James Bay Treaty established when the large hydroelectric projects were developed on their lands about thirty years ago. One of the band councils had the wisdom to recognize that their band members would be healthier living in the forest in the old way than sitting around the reservation eating potato chips and getting fat. They decided that in order to receive any treaty money, a family would have to live off the land in nomadic hunting camps; for this they would receive ten dollars per day per family member. Members of that band would go out in the fall to the forest, build hunting camps, and live there through the winter, returning to the reservation in the spring (when the blackflies came out) for summer holidays.

Since the mercury in the water system that serves the Swampy Cree concentrates in larger fish and then in fish-eating birds, we were trying to determine how often the people ate fish, game, fowl, and fish-eating birds. When the dietician asked them how often they ate such foods, the response was essentially "as often as possible." When the concept of an average weekly consumption was communicated through the interpreter, it turned out that on average, they ate some kind of meat (animal flesh) about three times a week.

It was striking to the medical team how much healthier the members of that band were compared to the members of a neighboring band who spent all year on the reservation. For me, the lesson was that human beings are designed to eat meat about three times a week, and that when we eat a meat-based diet, we get into trouble.

The second trip that changed my thinking about diet was to China in 1985. When we visited the largest hospital in Beijing, the capital (then a city of eight million), the resident in the intensive care unit proudly presented the case of a man who had experienced a heart attack; apparently, heart attacks were quite rare in that hospital. In response to my question about how often they saw such cases, she said with pride, "Oh, of course we are a major referral center, but we see thirty-seven such patients per year." I was floored. In those days we saw, in our small city of 350,000, about a hundred patients with heart attacks every month.

It turns out that in North America we have about six hundred heart attacks per 100,000 population annually, compared to sixty per 100,000 in China. People of Chinese origin who live in North America, however, have just as many heart attacks as do other Americans. This means that the major difference is environmental, not genetic: the main difference is diet.

The North American diet is based on the notion that the meat is the star of the meal, and we tend to think of the vegetables as unimportant side dishes, such as flavorless peas, carrots, and string beans. We therefore spend little time or energy on the preparation of vegetables.

Indeed, our food-delivery chain is so strong that we can simply buy groceries, heat them, and eat them. I call this approach "heated groceries," as opposed to cuisine. It's time for us to adjust our thinking in order to influence our dietary habits to prevent atherosclerosis. We need to control our intake of saturated fats and cholesterol (primarily from animal food sources), put more emphasis on increasing our total dietary fiber intake, and place vegetables, among other high-fiber foods, at the top of the list in meal planning.

To make a healthy diet enjoyable, it really helps to switch from heated groceries to cuisine!

Reducing Cholesterol and Saturated Fats

A diet too high in saturated fats may raise the blood cholesterol level and increase the risk of heart disease. To reduce the amount of cholesterol and saturated fats in our diet, we need to:

- Reduce our intake of foods high in dietary cholesterol such as animal flesh, butter, and cheese, and eliminate egg yolks
- Reduce our total intake of saturated fats, which means avoiding high-fat dairy products and high-fat meats
- Read labels of packaged foods: choose items favoring monounsaturated and polyunsaturated fats, and avoid trans fats (explained later)

- Increase our overall consumption of whole-grain breads, cereals, fresh fruits, and vegetables to enhance our fiber intake; a diet high in soluble fiber helps lower cholesterol.

Although chicken and fish are lower in saturated fats than red meat, the cholesterol content is the same among various types of animal flesh: about 100 mg (a whole day's target intake) per four-ounce serving. Therefore the word *meat* here refers to animal flesh of all kinds, not just to "red" meat.

Saturated Fats

Dietary fat is found in foods that come from plants and animals. Fat is an essential part of the diet and a major source of energy; however, the typical North American diet tends to be too high in total fats (approximately 39 percent of total calories consumed). Reducing the total amount of dietary fat to about 30 percent of the total daily calories, with 10 percent coming from saturated fats, complies with the current dietary recommendations for the NCEP Step 1 diet; a Step 2 diet, as we have seen, calls for fewer than 200 mg of cholesterol per day, with 20 percent or fewer calories from fat and 10 percent from saturated fat.

Saturated fats occur in the largest amounts in meat and dairy products. Reading food labels has become increasingly important since items such as coconut, palm, and palm-kernel oils (also saturated fats or hydrogenated vegetable oils, that is, trans fats) may appear in some processed items. Popcorn in movie theaters can be loaded with saturated fat or trans fats, although some chains are now using canola oil.

The chemical process that converts liquid (unsaturated) fats into solid (saturated) fats is called *hydrogenation*. This produces trans fats, which are particularly harmful. Be aware of the fine print on food labels in terms of the percentage of hydrogenation, or the percentage of trans fats. Avoid trans fats as much as possible. This means avoiding hydrogenated vegetable oil, or shortening, and foods cooked in it.

Margarine

Switching from butter to margarine helps, but it is important to understand that the hydrogenated fats used to make margarine more solid are high in trans fats, which are harmful; bad margarines are worse than butter. It is important to choose a non-hydrogenated margarine high in polyunsaturated and monounsaturated fats, and low in saturated fats. Some of the best margarines are based on canola oil, which is high in monounsaturated fats and contains omega-3 fats. It is best to choose a margarine with "non-hydrogenated" and/or "zero trans fats" on the label.

Oils for Cooking and Salads

Choosing the healthiest oils for your kitchen can be tricky. Olive oil tastes good and is high in monounsaturated fats, so it is a good choice for salads, but it breaks down when heated, with production of trans fatty acids. Canola oil takes the heat better and is a better choice for cooking methods such as stir-frying. Peanut oil is probably even better, but stirring quickly to keep below the smoke point of the oil may be the key. Remember, though, that even "good" oils are still fifty calories per teaspoon, so quantity is important. It helps to use a nonstick wok—keep a bowl of water handy so you can splash a teaspoon or so of water into the wok to make steam if things are sticking.

A useful trick for providing the flavor of fat with a very small quantity of oil is to use a few drops of sesame oil in dishes such as vegetarian chili that seem a bit austere without any oil.

Increasing Whole Grains

An important part of the Cretan Mediterranean diet is whole grains; compared to refined carbohydrates, such as table sugar and white bread, whole grains not only reduce the risk of cancer but also lower cholesterol and improve insulin resistance. Our diet should include whole-grain bread and cereals, whole-grain pasta, and brown rice as much as is reasonable.

An important way of looking at foods made from grains involves the glycemic index, which deals with how quickly foods are converted to sugar. On a scale of 0 to 100, table sugar is 100; white bread, white rice, and potatoes are about 80; brown rice about 60; and whole-grain pasta about 20. A website useful for looking up foods to see where they fit is www.glycemicindex.com.

Increasing Vegetables

A good place to start learning how to cook meals that are based on vegetables is with the Chinese culture, since the Chinese have a five-thousand-year head start on most North Americans. (Recipes still exist for what the emperor was served on his birthday thousands of years ago.) We can go to vegetarian, Chinese, and Indian restaurants, find vegetarian dishes we enjoy, and pay attention to how they were prepared. We can purchase a wok and experiment with a selection of wok and vegetarian cookbooks.

Learning to prepare vegetable dishes with star quality will make it easier to reduce our intake of meat. We can learn to make meals based on tasty, interesting dishes that include such vegetables as zucchini, bok choy, celery, onions, green and red peppers, ginger, garlic, green onions, and sometimes a small portion of meat (two or three ounces per person). "A Guide to Healthy Meals" at the end of the book includes instructions and recipes for such dishes.

For most of us, reducing meat intake to two ounces a day is a major change; while we're learning to do this, it may be easier to go meatless every other day and keep to four ounces total on meat days. (A four-ounce serving of meat is about the size of a deck of cards, or the size of the palm of your hand.) Fish is better than chicken, which is better than beef, but remember that meat is anything with eyes, a face, or a mother; anything that walks, swims, crawls, or flies!

Treating Cholesterol with Drugs

The best way to make sure that treatment is appropriate is to base the treatment on an individual's risk level, rather than on his or her cholesterol level. For people with several risk factors, or for people with identified blockage in the arteries to the heart, brain, or legs, it is definitely better to treat cholesterol with drugs than to withhold drug treatment. For people who have mildly or moderately elevated cholesterol but normal arteries and no other risk factors, it may be appropriate to use diet, exercise, and soluble fiber.

Secondary Prevention

There is no longer any doubt that individuals who have already experienced a heart attack or who have angina (chest pain or tightness when you hurry or lift something heavy) benefit from cholesterol-lowering drugs. Statin drugs—which reduce blood cholesterol levels by inhibiting a key enzyme involved in the biosynthesis of cholesterol—reduce heart attacks by 40 percent in six years, or better. They also reduce stroke in individuals with coronary disease by about 30 percent. It is very likely that they will reduce stroke substantially among others who have experienced a small warning stroke or a stroke; studies are under way to address that question.

If you have a high cholesterol level and have symptoms from your arteries such as angina, pain in the calf brought on by walking and relieved by rest (intermittent claudication), or small warning strokes (TIAs), these are the risks for drug treatment: over the next six years, overall mortality risk is reduced by 30 percent, and the risk of needing a bypass operation is reduced by 37 percent; the risk of stroke is also reduced significantly, and there is no increased risk of cancer, violent death, or other causes of death.

The risk of a significant adverse reaction from a cholesterol-lowering drug is about 1:1,000, and that risk can be virtually eliminated by having a blood test to measure the blood levels of enzymes from the muscles and liver; if a problem shows up and you stop the drug, the problem will almost always clear up, unless the blood test was done too late. (It would be reasonable to have a blood test about a month after starting medication; if that is normal, repeat blood testing is probably not necessary.) A risk of 1:1,000 is 0.1 percent; subtract that from 40 percent and you still have a net benefit of 39.99 percent—in other words, the benefit outweighs the risk by about 400 to 1.

Cholesterol-Lowering Drug Treatments

Five main kinds of drug treatments exist for adverse lipid profiles: bile-acid sequestrant resins such as cholestyramine and colestipol, which work by binding bile salts, which are made from cholesterol, in the bowel, so they are eliminated); ezetimibe, which reduces absorption of cholesterol; niacin (a B vitamin); fibrate drugs such as gemfibrozil, bezafibrate, and fenofibrate; and the statin drugs, which inhibit cholesterol synthesis in the liver by inhibiting an enzyme, HMG CoA reductase—these are often called *HMG CoA Reductase Inhibitors*, which is an awful mouthful, so I prefer to call them *statins*, since that ending identifies them all. Lovastatin, simvastatin, pravastatin, fluvastatin, atorvastatin, and rosuvastatin are available so far, and undoubtedly more are coming.

To choose the best treatment for you, it is important to know whether you have a high total cholesterol with normal triglycerides (TG) and HDL ("good" cholesterol), or a high cholesterol with high triglycerides and low HDL: the treatments are different.

For high cholesterol with normal TG and HDL, the statins are most effective, and adding a bile-acid sequestrant powder or a new drug that reduces absorption of cholesterol, ezetimibe, will increase the benefit. For high or even normal cholesterol with high TG and low HDL, the most effective treatment is niacin; however some people can't take niacin, and for them the fibrates are the best alternative. For high-risk people with low HDL it is probably best to combine a statin with niacin or a fibrate.

Bile-Acid Sequestrants—and an Inexpensive Alternative

Every time you eat, there is a reflex emptying of the gallbladder, which pours bile salts into the upper intestine to help with fat absorption. The bile salts normally are reabsorbed by the intestine, go to the liver, and get stored back in the gallbladder. The liver makes bile salts from cholesterol, so if you prevent them from being reabsorbed and evacuate them with your bowel movements, the liver has to take cholesterol out of the bloodstream to make new bile salts—thus lowering your total cholesterol level.

That is how the bile-acid sequestrants cholestyramine and

colestipol work. They are resin powders that you mix with water or juice and drink before a meal. The bile salts bind to them and get eliminated, so they lower cholesterol levels by about 10–15 percent, if you can take enough. To achieve that benefit requires about four doses a day, which can be difficult to take. The powders have a gritty texture that some people don't like, and they also tend to cause problems with bloating and constipation.

Because of these adverse effects, many individuals have unfortunately chosen the easier approach of taking a tablet of statin at bedtime. I say "unfortunately" because there is a much greater lowering of cholesterol when statins are taken along with bile-acid sequestrants, but the adverse effects and the cost (about a hundred dollars per month for bile-acid sequestrants compared to about fifty dollars per month for statins) have led to underutilization of these effective treatments.

We did a study in our research unit that found a way around these problems. If you'll recall, like bile-acid sequestrants, soluble fiber binds bile salts. Psyllium mucilloid (e.g., Metamucil), which is about the most concentrated form of soluble fiber, is often used to treat constipation, so it seemed likely to help with the problem of constipation caused by the sequestrants. In fact, if you take a half-and-half mixture of colestipol and psyllium (half a teaspoon of each, mixed into juice or water) before each meal, you will get a nearly double reduction of cholesterol with fewer side effects. An additional benefit is a marked reduction in cost, since psyllium is cheap: about thirteen dollars for a two-pound jar that will last about six months. Mixing it half and half with colestipol or cholestyramine reduces the cost by almost half (25).

Niacin: Great Stuff, but Tricky to Take

Niacin, or vitamin B_3, is the most cost-effective way to treat problems with cholesterol. In addition to raising HDL and lowering triglycerides, niacin reduces total cholesterol, and it is the best of the cholesterol treatments at lowering a new risk factor called lipoprotein(a) or Lp(a) (pronounced "ell pee little a"). This is a lipoprotein that seems to interact with fibrinogen, a clotting factor, and high levels are a risk factor even in people who have normal cholesterol levels. It is not yet measured routinely in most laboratories, so it is hard to know if you have a problem with it, but lowering it is a particular benefit of niacin.

Niacin is also cheap, available over the counter for about ten dollars per month. So why isn't it used more often?

The problem is that for the first few days, it produces very impressive flushing of the skin, and many people refuse to take it after the first dose. As a result, many doctors have unfortunately given up on it.

The flushing is not harmful. It goes away after five days at full doses in most people, and studies show that about 80 percent of people can take niacin; the challenge is to persist. The flush can be truly amazing: once when I took niacin for a research project, I turned red as a beet, I felt hot and prickly all over, and my eyes burned a bit for about a half hour after each dose for the first three days. Then it settled down.

It helps to take the niacin after meals rather than on an empty stomach. Some people find it easier to take a small dose at first and increase the dose gradually. Try starting with 100 mg, or half a 500 mg tablet three times a day after meals, and then increase it about every third day until you are up to 500 mg three times a day. Some people take a gram (1,000 mg) or more three times a day, but I think 500 mg three times a day will achieve most of the benefit with less risk of the two main adverse effects: niacin can aggravate gout and diabetes.

PREVENT NIACIN FLUSHING WITH ASA

The flushing from niacin is due to release of a prostaglandin called pGD2, which widens blood-vessel channels. Since ASA (acetylsalicylic acid, or aspirin) inhibits the synthesis of prostaglandins, it is quite effective for preventing flushing if you take it three times a day (or use a slow-release ASA) for several days before starting the niacin. (After you are on the full dose of niacin and the flushing has settled down, you will be able to reduce the ASA to one a day.)

Niacin is the most effective, cheapest, and safest of the treatments for cholesterol. It should be used a lot more than it is. If you can, you should put up with the flushing for a few days until it settles down. A small proportion of individuals simply can't take niacin, and for them, drugs are often required.

SLOW-RELEASE OR "NONFLUSH" NIACIN

Beware the pharmacist who suggests slow-release or nonflush niacin. Ralph Stern and I showed that most slow-release niacin is metabolized in a way that makes it ineffective for reducing cholesterol and more toxic to the liver (26). Niacinamide is also ineffective for cholesterol. The only safe and effective slow-release niacin that I know of is Niaspan, which costs more than a dollar a day. If you have low HDL and can't take niacin using the measures just described (or you can't be bothered with the struggle), Niaspan is probably a good choice.

Fibrates

If you can't take niacin and you have high triglycerides with low HDL, your best bet is a fibrate. Available options include clofibrate, gemfibrozil, fenofibrate, and bezafibrate. These drugs probably all increase the risk of gallbladder problems a bit, but if you are a high-risk individual with vascular disease, the benefit clearly outweighs the risk: which would you rather have—a stroke, or a gallbladder operation?

When statins (which inhibit cholesterol synthesis in the liver) are combined with fibrates, the risk of mild liver problems goes up to about 1 percent, and mild muscle problems may occur in 5–10 percent of individuals; this level of risk is still much lower than the level of benefit (about a 40 percent reduction in risk in high-risk individuals), so the ratio of risk to benefit for people at high risk is strongly in favor of using them. It is prudent to take the precaution of having a blood test about a month after starting the combination to make sure that you aren't in the 1 percent. The best frequency of retesting while on this combination isn't established, but probably once or twice a year would be enough if the first test is normal (or sooner if you're unwell; the symptoms would likely resemble a flu, with achy weak muscles).

For now, the fibrates gemfibrozil, fenofibrate, and bezafibrate appear to be about equally effective and safe; there are no good drug-to-drug comparisons available. One advantage of fenofibrate and bezafibrate is their once-a-day preparation, which is more convenient. However, fenofibrate raises the levels of total homocysteine by about 40 percent and bezafibrate by about 15 percent, and they can aggravate kidney failure, so vitamin therapy for homocysteine may be needed and kidney function may require monitoring. Gemfibrozil is less likely to cause high homocysteine or kidney impairment, but it has significant problems with drug interactions: it was an interaction between gemfibrozil and cerivastatin (Baycol) that was partly responsible for the severe muscle problems that caused cerivastatin to be withdrawn from the market. (Muscle problems from statins are discussed in Chapter 9.)

Statins

The statin drugs have revolutionized the prevention of vascular disease. They work by reducing the amount of cholesterol that your liver makes, which causes the liver to make more receptors for LDL (low-density lipoprotein) and draw more cholesterol out of the bloodstream, in addition to making less. As we have seen, they reduce formation of cholesterol by inhibiting in the liver an enzyme called HMG CoA reductase, a key enzyme early in the formation of cholesterol. The drugs include lovastatin, simvastatin, fluvastatin, pravastatin, atorvastatin, and rosuvastatin. Most people tolerate them very well; only about 1 in 15,000 will have significant liver problems, which can be detected early with a blood test, and the problem goes away if you stop the drug. About 1–3 percent of people will have an increase in blood levels of liver enzymes, reflecting not liver damage but a change in enzyme kinetics. Occasionally, diarrhea is a problem.

In addition to large studies that show a decrease in coronary events with use of statins, a number of smaller studies show that these drugs result in improvement of the coronary arteries in some individuals and slow down the rate at which they get worse in virtually all individuals. Ultrasound studies of the carotid arteries also show regression of atherosclerosis with effective LDL cholesterol reduction and increases in HDL.

Interestingly, events such as heart attacks decrease much faster than does plaque in the arteries. It is thought this difference is because lowering cholesterol makes plaques less likely to rupture and improves the function of the endothelium (the lining of the artery), which is involved in spasm of the arteries and the formation of clots. Another reason may be reduced inflammation in the arteries by mechanisms unrelated to cholesterol lowering.

Statins are expensive, and understanding their value is tricky: the cheapest drug isn't the best buy, because it doesn't lower cholesterol as well.

Pitfalls of Drug Treatment for Cholesterol

There are three main groups for whom cholesterol-lowering drugs are inappropriately used. The first are people who take statins who are at relatively low risk because they are young, with no other risk factors, and only a mild or moderate elevation of cholesterol. That condition, in which the use of statins is called *primary prevention*, is probably more suited to nondrug therapy, since the risk is fairly low for a long time. The second group is women at risk of pregnancy, who should not take any drugs for cholesterol except bile-acid sequestrants. They can instead work for years with dietary restriction of cholesterol and saturated fats, weight loss, exercise, and soluble fiber, and consider taking drugs only when the risk levels are higher. In that situation, there is probably some inappropriate overtreatment of cholesterol.

I believe that a much commoner problem is inappropriate undertreatment of cholesterol in individuals who have known vascular disease. This applies to two groups of people. In the first group are people who have had a coronary bypass operation, or a balloon angioplasty of their leg arteries or coronary arteries, but are not being treated for their cholesterol problem at all. When I ask them why on earth they are still eating eggs and not doing anything about their lipids, they say the doctor told them their arteries were cured. That approach is crazy; I expect that what those people heard is not what their doctors meant to say. Surgeons can operate on a few inches of artery here and there, but a body has miles of arteries to keep open. Repeat surgery is much more difficult and risky, in part because of scar tissue, and artery disease will recur much sooner without attention to all the risk factors—smoking being the most important.

The second group includes people whose cholesterol is being treated with too low a dose of medication. In some cases the problem is neglected because the cholesterol level isn't very high. Often doctors seem to think that once the decision has been made to prescribe a drug, the problem is dealt with. What is really needed is treatment of the cholesterol to a target level that is quite low. For someone with artery trouble, it is not okay to have the average cholesterol level for a North American; the goal is a nice low Chinese cholesterol level, meaning about half what the average is in North America. So people with vascular disease and "normal" cholesterol levels probably need to be treated, and the treatment needs to be to a lower target level than most doctors think. A desirable LDL below 75 mg/dl (2 mmol/L), or a ratio of total cholesterol to HDL of less than 3, would be more effective than treating to "normal" levels. Most guideline committees are discussing even lower target levels, based on recent studies.

The Bottom Line

If you have a high risk of vascular disease, you should be trying to improve your lipid profile. You should take a positive attitude; think in terms of learning to make a healthy eating pattern delicious. Reduce your intake of cholesterol and saturated fats, learn how to make the Cretan Mediterranean diet enjoyable, increase your intake of soluble fiber, maintain a lean weight, and exercise to raise HDL.

If you already have artery disease, or if you have a very high risk level because of family history or a combination of risk factors, drugs that lower cholesterol are indicated, and the benefits clearly outweigh the risks. There is no point in waiting a year to see if diet works for you; diet is about nonfasting (after-meal) fat, not about fasting lipids. Serious liver problems caused by cholesterol-lowering drugs are very rare, and for most people that experience muscle problems from statins, there are ways around that problem.

8
How to Control
High Blood Pressure

Arterial hypertension, usually shortened to *hypertension*, is the medical term for high blood pressure; it does not imply nervous tension or stress. For most people with hypertension, the problem is mild, there is no underlying cause other than a tendency for high blood pressure that runs in the family, and the problem can often be managed for many years without drugs. Also, individuals who require drugs for blood pressure can often reduce the amount of medication that is required by improving their non-drug therapy. It is, however, very important not to set yourself up for disappointment by hoping that you can avoid "evil" drugs if you just behave well enough. Yes, there are adverse effects from drugs, but you have to keep in perspective the balance of the risks: if your blood pressure is high enough, or if you have other risk factors besides hypertension, your risk without drugs is much higher than the risks associated with drugs.

Treating High Blood Pressure without Drugs

Effective measures to improve blood pressure without drugs include weight loss, exercise, and avoidance of substances that aggravate blood pressure.

Substances That Aggravate Blood Pressure

The most important substance to avoid is salt, so there's a whole section on it later. Other things you put in your mouth that will aggravate blood pressure include alcohol, licorice, decongestant medications and amphetamine relatives such as appetite suppressants and pep pills, birth-control pills, and nonsteroidal anti-inflammatory drugs.

ALCOHOL

Despite favorable publicity lately for red wine under the rubric "the French paradox," there are problems with too much alcohol. Besides the obvious social costs, health issues such as liver failure, and the terrible toll associated with drinking and driving, too much alcohol will raise your blood pressure. The entire explanation for the connection isn't entirely clear, but one problem is that alcohol releases adrenaline from the adrenal gland.

Over the ages, we have pretty much established what constitutes a serving of alcohol: one glass of wine, one beer, and one highball each contains about the same amount. It seems that, compared to no alcohol intake, one drink per day is associated with a lower risk of heart attacks and strokes, but more than two drinks per day will raise blood pressure; some people seem to react more to alcohol than do others. I learned about this from a patient whose hypertension was not well controlled for years, despite his taking several different kinds of medication for a total of about seven pills per day. He came into our clinic one day with a normal pressure despite stopping all but a half tablet daily of one of the pills; he explained that he had never admitted that he was drinking a quart of whiskey a day, and when he stopped drinking his pressure was so low that he had to stop most of his pills.

Some people can't stop after the first drink; if this sounds like you, quitting completely may be the best (or only) solution. For others, it helps to have alternatives for the second and subsequent drinks, especially for social occasions. Try iced tea, diet pop with a wedge of lime, ginger beer, and low-alcohol beers with less than 1 percent alcohol (if you chill the beer and glass well, these are surprisingly good).

DECONGESTANT MEDICATIONS

Nose sprays and cold remedies that contain decongestants such as phenylpropanolamine or pseudo-ephedrine, pep pills such as phenylpropanolamine, weight-loss remedies that work by suppressing appetite, and some street drugs such as speed (methylamphetamine, crystal meth) and cocaine raise blood pressure either by releasing noradrenaline and adrenaline from nerve endings in sympathetic nerves (part of the autonomic nervous system), or by simulating release of these hormones, which affect the same receptors on the blood vessels and the heart. Phenypropanolamine has been taken off the market in the United States for this reason, but it is still available in some countries, and it may be contained in some herbal remedies or drugs purchased over the internet. Although in most people with mild hypertension an occasional dose of decongestant may not usually be a problem, there can be significant difficulties for people with severe hypertension or with prolonged use. In inner-city hospitals, cocaine and crystal meth are important causes of brain hemorrhages in young people.

One patient who taught me about decongestants was a young lawyer who had been using decongestant nose spray for several years. Whenever he tried to stop the nose spray, his nasal congestion got worse (rebound nasal congestion is very common), so he had worked up to nine doses per day. Within two weeks of stopping the nose spray, his blood pressure was down from 180/120 to 160/100. It can be very difficult to stop nose sprays, because of the rebound—you have to realize that it will be a problem for two or three days; sometimes corticosteroid nose sprays such as beclomethasone are very helpful.

For people with seasonal allergies such as tree pollens in the spring, grasses in the summer, and ragweed in the fall, or for people with allergies all year round (house mites in dust, moulds in house plants, etc.), a better alternative to decongestants is non-sedating antihistamines that do *not* contain decongestants, topical steroid nose sprays such as beclomethasone, and eyedrops such as sodium chromoglycate.

Ask your family doctor or your pharmacist for advice about over-the-counter preparations if you are unsure.

BIRTH-CONTROL PILLS

Occasionally, birth-control pills can cause high blood pressure. This seems to be less common with lower-dose pills, particularly with lower doses of progesterone, which is probably the problem, rather than estrogen. The blood pressure can take three to four months to rise and several months to drop again, so don't be thrown off if your blood pressure seems to stay up for a month or two after you stop the pill. If stopping the pill makes no difference after a few months, and treatment of your high blood pressure is successful, it is probably reasonable to cautiously restart the pill with close supervision for a few months. If stopping the pill seems to make a big difference, you probably need to stay off it.

Take heart in the facts: although the failure rate of the pill is slightly lower than that of barrier methods (0.0023 percent per year versus 0.028 percent above age twenty-five), the two approaches accomplish a similar result if they are used properly. Using foam along with a condom or diaphragm will reduce the risk further, and barrier methods have the additional benefit that they reduce the risk of sexually transmitted diseases such as HIV. Condoms are therefore advisable anyway for people in a new relationship. For stable monogamous couples, foam and diaphragm are often a reasonable approach.

NONSTEROIDAL ANTI-INFLAMMATORY DRUGS

Nonsteroidal anti-inflammatory drugs (NSAIDs, often called arthritis pills) work in part by inhibiting the formation of prostaglandins, some of which are important causes of inflammation. They are mainly used, therefore, in inflammatory conditions such as rheumatoid arthritis. These drugs also relieve pain—some more than others. They are often used for back pain, headache, menstrual cramps, and other conditions in which inflammation may be only a minor part of the problem.

The difficulty for people with high blood pressure is that some of the prostaglandins are also important in kidney function and in regulating blood pressure. They dilate arteries, so that blocking them can constrict arteries and impair kidney function. This leads to fluid retention, and worsening of blood pressure and heart failure.

For many individuals with osteoarthritis, or painful backs and necks, acetylsalicylic acid (ASA, or aspirin) or acetaminophen (e.g., Tylenol) may be just as effective as NSAIDs.

People who seem to need NSAIDs need to know that some cause less trouble than others. There has been a lot of publicity about Vioxx,

Celebrex, and their relations in the class called Cox 2 inhibitors, but all NSAIDs except sulindac aggravate hypertension. Sulindac has less effect on the kidneys and is less likely to aggravate blood pressure and heart failure, as some colleagues and I found (8). In some cases it may be necessary to consider gold therapy, methotrexate, or other "disease-modifying" drugs for rheumatoid arthritis; diuretics may help counteract the adverse effects of NSAIDs in individuals who require them.

People with gout may find allopurinol a useful preventive and colchicine a useful treatment, rather than relying on NSAIDs for prevention. Colchicine, which can be used even in kidney failure and heart failure, is an old remedy that many doctors are unfamiliar with, so you may need to raise the issue directly with your doctor.

LICORICE

Strange as it may seem, licorice contains a substance that causes salt and water retention and potassium loss. Its effects are similar to those of adrenal gland hormones such as aldosterone. A high intake of strong licorice can actually cause hypertension and potassium depletion, but this is rare: in the first ten years of operation of my Hypertension Clinic, only three of some four thousand patients with difficult hypertension had licorice intake as the underlying cause. However, a large intake of licorice may aggravate preexisting hypertension. The odd piece of licorice is not a problem, but do not eat it daily in large quantities.

SALT

The normal North American diet contains about 10 to 20 grams of salt a day. Most of this is in the form of sodium chloride (ordinary table salt), but baking soda, sodium bicarbonate, sodium nitrate (butcher's salt), monosodium glutamate, and other sodium salts turn up in many surprising forms.

People who routinely salt their food at the table before tasting it are usually eating more than 20 grams of salt a day, and people who salt their food after tasting it are usually eating about 10 grams of salt a day. This means that people who add salt at the table are eating ten to twenty times as much salt as they need. Amazingly, your body requires only *half a gram* of salt a day.

If you have high blood pressure, it is important to reduce your salt intake, because if you consume a lot of salt, your body will retain water in order to maintain the correct salt level in your bloodstream. This will not only raise your blood pressure, but also cause you to have more adverse effects from diuretic medications (sometimes called fluid pills or water pills, because they remove fluids from the body).

Most diuretic medications, such as hydrochlorothiazide, work initially by removing salt and water from the body through the kidneys. After about six weeks, the water balance within the body is restored, and the medication then works by dilating the small artery branches called arterioles.

As long as you are on a potassium-wasting diuretic such as hydrochlorothiazide or furosemide (Lasix and other brands), you have a tendency to lose potassium in the urine, and because the kidney exchanges potassium ions for sodium ions, the more sodium you eat, the more potassium you lose. A shortage of potassium in the cells causes aching and cramping in the muscles and is often not detected by a blood test, which checks the potassium level in the bloodstream. About 90 percent of the potassium in the body is contained within the cells, and it is quite common to have a normal blood level in the face of a significant depletion of potassium within the cells (27). (See Chapter 11 for more information about how to manage potassium depletion.)

Although some researchers focus on distinguishing between people who are salt sensitive and those who are salt resistant, it seems likely that people who can get away with eating salt have milder blood pressure, and those whose blood pressure goes up with salt are people with more severe high blood pressure, with thickening of the small artery branches (arterioles). I believe that most people with hypertension will benefit from salt restriction; this is particularly true for the elderly, and for people with hypertension that is difficult to control.

Salting one's food is mainly a habit, but it is also the consequence of a change in taste sensation that occurs when one eats a lot of salt. The more salt we eat, the more taste buds in our tongue shrivel, so after a while, we can't taste the salt that is already in the foods. The good news is that if we markedly reduce our salt intake, the taste buds will grow back, and we can then taste the salt already in foods. This means we don't miss salt as much as we think we will. Fortunately, it only takes about three weeks for the taste buds to grow back.

The goal is to reduce salt intake to two to three grams of salt per day.

How to Reduce Salt Intake

To reduce the amount of salt we eat, we need to eliminate saltshakers from our routine, or replace the salt in shakers with a salt substitute called No-Salt, which is a mixture of potassium salts (not to be used by those who have had high potassium levels, or who are in kidney failure). We also need to markedly reduce our intake of foods that contain a lot of salt, like canned soups and cured meats. A cup of tomato soup contains a gram of salt, one cup of tomato juice contains half a gram, a slice of back bacon contains half a gram, and a slice of ham contains nearly a gram. Salted chips, in particular, are extremely salty. (In fact, we shouldn't eat chips at all: they contain saturated fats and trans fats, and so much fat is soaked into them they are ten calories each.) In general, we should avoid cured meats, canned soups, and canned vegetables (a cup of canned corn contains nearly half a gram of salt, whereas the same amount of fresh or frozen corn contains virtually none).

Pickles are a particular problem. One dill pickle contains two grams of salt, and so does an equivalent amount of most kinds of pickles. That's a whole day's intake! One can make pickles without salt, but a simpler alternative is to slice tomatoes, cucumbers, beets, or other vegetables into a bowl and pour some vinegar over them.

There are many other ways to make food tasty without using salt, for instance, by adding lemon juice, lime juice, vinegar, herbs, spices, pepper, hot pepper, ginger, garlic, green onions, green peppers, curry powder, or commercial salt substitutes such as No-Salt. Celery salt, garlic salt, half salt, sea salt, or other products that contain sodium are traps to watch out for, since they still contain a lot of salt. In place of salty chips, try popcorn sprinkled with Cajun spice or some other salt-free flavoring. In tomato juice, try some lime juice, vinegar, and/or tabasco sauce.

Mustard powder is a useful spice. A teaspoon of mustard powder added to oil and vinegar with some Italian spices makes a salt-free salad dressing that has some tang to it. Similarly, a teaspoon of mustard powder with some barbecue spices, hot pepper flakes, chopped fresh ginger, and red wine makes a tasty marinade and barbecue sauce. (Commercial barbecue sauce has about two grams of salt to a cup; other commercial sauces such as steak sauce, ketchup, and so on are also to be avoided.)

It is best to make a clean break with salt. That way, taste buds will grow back in fairly quickly. You will know you are winning in about three weeks, when some foods you used to salt begin to taste too salty.

Drugs that Treat High Blood Pressure

A number of different kinds of drugs work to lower high blood pressure. They include medications that get rid of salt and water (diuretics), drugs that dilate arteries (vasodilators), and drugs that block the effect of adrenaline on the heart (beta-blockers) and arteries (alpha-blockers). Often a small dose of two or more drugs with different actions works well, achieving a greater reduction in blood pressure and with less adverse effects, because the dose of each does not need to be as high as it would if used alone.

Diuretics

The commonest and cheapest drug for treating high blood pressure is hydrochlorothiazide, a drug that is particularly effective in the elderly and, as we will see, in people with African ancestors. It is a member of a family called the *thiazide diuretics* and acts first as a diuretic; after six weeks or so, its main effect is to relax the small artery branches, the arterioles. The main issue with this drug is determining the correct dose: for most individuals a dose of 12.5 mg daily is enough, and for some individuals 12.5 mg every other day. In the heat of summer, or in hot climates, when one perspires more, the dose sometimes needs to be reduced. Hydrochlorothiazide is usually available in tablets of 25 mg or more, so half of the smallest tablet is the optimal dose.

Too much of the drug can aggravate gout, diabetes, cholesterol, and depletion of potassium, magnesium, and other ions, so higher doses are not better; stick to 12.5 mg. This is a nuisance in that the tablets have to be broken, but taking the drug is extra cheap because of that: a month's treatment costs less than a dollar, plus the dispensing fee. This is one example of a drug for which a one-month supply makes no sense at all: the dispensing fee probably will cost more than a year's supply.

Thiazide diuretics, in addition to the problems just mentioned, can in some cases raise blood levels of calcium. For people who experience rashes caused by exposure to the sun (photosensitivity), these can usually be managed with hat, sunscreen, and sun avoidance.

But the main problem—and it is tricky—is potassium depletion. Because most elderly persons need a bit of diuretic for control, hydrochlorothiazide is a very important drug, and for that reason I later devote a whole section to avoiding problems with depletion of potassium and other ions that are lost when diuretics are used inappropriately.

Similar drugs include chlorthalidone and indapamide, but there are problems with both: chlorthalidone comes only in doses that are too high, and it is so long acting, it tends to cause more problems with potassium depletion. Indapamide is claimed to cause less problems with cholesterol than does hydrochlorothiazide, but a study we did showed no difference, and it costs a lot more. For most individuals who need a diuretic, a low dose of hydrochlorothiazide is the best buy.

Beta-Blockers

Beta-blockers block one of the two kinds of adrenaline receptor (a structure on the surface of cells that responds to adrenaline), the beta receptors. Beta receptors are of two types, beta-1 and beta-2. Stimulating beta-1 receptors causes the heart to speed up and beat more forcefully. Stimulating beta-2 receptors causes the bronchi, the large air tubes in the lungs, to dilate, and causes the arteries that go to muscles to dilate, so the blood flow to the muscles increases. Beta-2 stimulation also has metabolic effects such as an increase in insulin release, and effects on cholesterol and sugar metabolism.

In general, these functions are useful for emergencies such as running away from a saber-tooth tiger; that's why our ancestors who had them survived and passed them on to us. Unfortunately, these reactions may not serve us well in a stressful urban environment.

Beta-blockers lower blood pressure mainly by blocking beta-1 receptors; they keep the heart calm and slow even when we are excited or upset. Blocking beta-2 receptors causes adverse effects—for example, beta-blockers that block these receptors aggravate asthma by tending to constrict the bronchi, aggravate cold extremities, and reduce exercise capacity by limiting skin and muscle blood flow; they also aggravate diabetes and cholesterol metabolism.

For this reason, beta-blockers that mainly affect beta-1 receptors tend to have fewer adverse effects than do those that block both beta-1 and beta-2 receptors (nonselective beta-blockers). A third class of beta-blockers block beta-1 receptors and stimulate beta-2 receptors; these drugs are said to have "intrinsic sympathomimetic activity," or ISA. In theory they should work better than the other beta-blockers, but they have their own problems; some of them concentrate more in the brain and in high doses can cause vivid dreams, tremors, anxiety, and sometimes cramps.

Nonselective beta-blockers include propranolol, timolol, and nadolol; relatively selective beta-blockers are atenolol and metoprolol. Drugs with ISA include pindolol, oxprenolol, and acebutolol; of these, I prefer pindolol, because it is very long acting, stimulates beta-2 receptors more, and has less variable metabolism (less difference between individuals) than other beta-blockers have.

Alpha-Blockers

Alpha-blockers block the second of the two kinds of adrenaline receptor, the alpha receptors: the alpha-1 receptor when stimulated causes the arteries to constrict, and the alpha-2 receptor when stimulated inhibits the sympathetic nervous system.

Alpha-blockers by themselves are not recommended for treatment of hypertension, because they have proven less effective than other drugs, but they may be helpful in combination with other medications.

The main alpha-blockers in use selectively block the alpha-1 receptors; by preventing the arteries from constricting, they tend to help lower blood pressure. They also have beneficial effects on cholesterol and diabetes, and they are now commonly used for bladder symptoms from prostate gland enlargement. The main ones in use are prazosin, doxazosin, and terazosin. Compared with prazosin, the latter two are longer acting so can be taken less often, and they tend to cause less trouble with a faint feeling on standing. Doxazosin is the longest acting, and probably the best choice for that reason.

Vasodilators

HYDRALAZINE
The old standby among vasodilators—drugs that dilate arteries—is hydralazine, which has recently been resurrected for the treatment of heart failure, particularly for African Americans. When used alone, it causes the heart to speed up and tends to cause throbbing headaches, so it is usually used in combination with a beta-blocker. In large doses, in susceptible people, it can cause a form of lupus, with rashes, arthritis, and other problems. Some people metabolize hydralazine very slowly, so they may have problems at lower doses.

NITRATES
Nitroglycerine and the longer-acting nitrate drugs such as isosorbide dinitrate (Isordil) work in a different way from hydralazine; they release nitric oxide, a vasodilator substance produced in the artery lining. They are used mainly for the treatment of angina (chest pain or tightness when you hurry or lift something heavy) and would seldom be used to treat hypertension, except perhaps as a nitroglycerine patch applied in the emergency room in an acute situation.

CALCIUM-CHANNEL ANTAGONISTS
Calcium-channel antagonists, or calcium-channel blockers, dilate arteries by interfering with the channels that permit calcium to enter cells; they are useful for both hypertension and angina. Drugs in the class called *dihydropyridines*, the largest group, tend to be the best at lowering blood pressure. Diltiazem is a somewhat weaker vasodilator in the peripheral arteries throughout the body, but it affects the coronary arteries and so may be better for angina. Verapamil is

a relatively weak drug for blood pressure and very expensive, but it is quite useful for heart-rhythm disturbances; its main problems are that it can cause constipation and may aggravate heart failure.

The main dihydropyridines are nifedipine, felodipine, amlodipine, nisoldipine, and nicardipine. Nifedipine and felodipine are quite short acting, and the slow-release pills that have been developed are only partially effective in correcting the problem of peaks and troughs in blood pressure. Some of the adverse effects such as flushing, headache, and ankle swelling appear to be related to high peak levels, so if you have problems with such side effects you may be better off with amlodipine, which is very long acting and therefore smoother.

Nifedipine is relatively expensive, but the best value is felodipine, and if it is causing too many side effects, amlodipine may be better. Nicardipine is very expensive and usually has to be taken several times a day, so it has little advantage.

A special problem occurs when dihydropyridines are taken with grapefruit juice (discussed in Chapter 10). Grapefruit contains substances that markedly reduce the metabolism of a number of drugs. We discovered the problem originally with felodipine, but the same thing occurs with nisoldipine and to a lesser extent with nifedipine. Felodipine blood levels go up on average about 300 percent with grapefruit juice, nisoldipine levels about 500 percent, and nifedipine levels about 30 percent. A number of important interactions occur between grapefruit and other drugs such as cyclosporine, terfenadine (an antihistamine), and propafenone; based on the known metabolism of warfarin and the cholesterol-lowering drugs such as lovastatin and simvastatin, it can be anticipated that they will also be affected by grapefruit juice.

Individualized Therapy for Hypertension

Finding the right treatment for hypertension for each individual turns out to be very important in managing not only potassium depletion, but also severe hypertension.

With rare exceptions, high blood pressure is related to the powerful hormone systems we need to survive that control salt and water. The exceptions include tumors of the inner part of the adrenal gland (the adrenal medulla) called *pheochromocytomas*, and a congenital narrowing of the aorta called *aortic coarctation*. In the more than ten thousand patients I have seen with difficult hypertension, there were only fifty-nine cases of pheochromocytoma, four adult cases of aortic coarctation, and nine due to licorice. Much commoner is high blood pressure due to kidney problems or to enlargement of the outer part of the adrenal gland (the adrenal cortex).

Measuring Blood Plasma Renin

To control high blood pressure in difficult cases, it is very important to figure out the cause, and the best way to sort out the cause is to measure the renin (a kidney enzyme) and aldosterone (an adrenal gland hormone) in the blood plasma (28, 29); this is most informative after the individual takes a dose of diuretic to stimulate the production of renin and aldosterone.

Figure 8.1 shows the central role of the kidney and adrenal gland in long-term regulation of body salt and water. They operate in a feedback loop that, when it works properly, is vital to survival. When it goes wrong, it causes high blood pressure. How it goes wrong is this: if the kidney senses that the body is too dry or the blood pressure is too low, it puts out renin, the enzyme that activates a precursor to angiotensin I, a short chain of amino acids. Angiotensin I is converted to angiotensin II by an enzyme called *angiotensin-converting enzyme* (ACE). Angiotensin II can raise blood pressure by itself because it constricts arteries, but there is a double whammy: it also goes to the outer part of the adrenal gland (the adrenal cortex) and causes the adrenal gland to release aldosterone. Aldosterone goes to the kidney, where it causes salt and water retention and excretion of potassium, magnesium, and other ions.

In individuals whose high blood pressure doesn't respond adequately to routine therapy, the key to getting the blood pressure under control is to sort out where the problem is in this feedback loop. If there is a problem with enlargement of the adrenal cortex, too much aldosterone is produced, causing salt and water retention and depletion of potassium, magnesium, and so on (primary hyperaldosteronism). In this situation, the salt and water retention suppresses the production of renin, so renin levels are abnormally low.

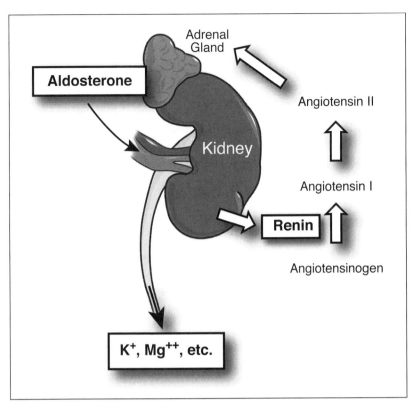

Figure 8.1 The use of plasma renin and aldosterone to pinpoint the physiological cause of high blood pressure when the feedback loop between the kidney and the adrenal cortex goes wrong, affecting the regulation of body salt and water

If the high blood pressure is due to a kidney problem—a blocked artery to one kidney, obstruction from kidney stones or scarring, multiple cysts, a tumor, or damage to the kidney from high blood pressure—the kidney makes too much renin, which inappropriately activates angiotensin and raises aldosterone (secondary hyperaldosteronism).

Most North Americans eat so much salt that the renin level in their blood plasma is usually quite low. For that reason, measuring the plasma renin without stimulation does not readily separate individuals with normal renin levels from those with low levels. Giving a dose of diuretic spreads out the range of renin levels, so it is possible to see the difference between low and normal (30). A similar approach uses a measurement of plasma renin and the sodium levels in a twenty-four-hour urine collection (31).

In individuals who have very low stimulated plasma renin levels after a dose of diuretic, hormones from the adrenal cortex, such as aldosterone, are usually responsible for the low renin. So these individuals don't need kidney tests (unless there is some other reason to do kidney tests, such as impaired kidney function, or blood or protein in the urine). Individuals with low stimulated plasma renin levels tend to respond better to diuretics, particularly potassium/magnesium-sparing diuretics, which prevent both magnesium and potassium depletion; they do not respond as well to angiotensin blockers or ACE inhibitors.

Individuals with high stimulated plasma renin levels need kidney tests, as they are much more likely to have a kidney problem as the cause of their high blood pressure; they respond much better to ACE inhibitors and angiotensin blockers. In some cases, when high blood pressure is caused by blockage of one of the kidney arteries, it may be necessary to restore blood flow to that kidney either by an angioplasty and stent—the insertion of a catheter and then of a balloon, inflated to stretch open the narrow segment of the artery, and insertion of a tube to keep the passage open—or a bypass operation.

By measuring stimulated plasma renin, we can now see, it is possible to guide not only the diagnosis but also the therapy in difficult cases of high blood pressure. (The routine we use is to measure plasma renin and aldosterone thirty minutes after an intravenous dose, or four hours after an oral dose, of furosemide (Lasix) 0.5 mg/kg.)

It should now be clear why figuring out the cause of high blood pressure in difficult cases is a critical step in treatment and control of the condition. In my more than four hundred cases of high blood pressure due to narrowing of the kidney arteries, for example, about half were controlled by using ACE (angiotensin-converting enzyme) inhibitors or angiotensin blockers (often along with a bit of diuretic and sometimes with the addition of other drugs), but about half have required a balloon dilation of the narrow artery (balloon angioplasty), and of those about 10 percent have needed kidney artery surgery (or removal of the kidney, if it could not be saved). Among individuals with high renin (kidney enzyme) levels, nine have turned out to have malignant kidney tumors, which were detected early enough for cure because the renin level was measured.

Hypertension among African Americans

An important issue in this respect is that two particular causes of hypertension are much more common among African Americans. Near where I work is a town called Buxton, which was a terminus of the Underground Railroad. Many of the people who live there are descendants of escaped slaves from the southern United States. Because of that coincidence, I have had a somewhat paradoxical and very instructive experience with special causes of hypertension in patients of African origin. Precisely because so few of the patients in our clinic (less than 1 percent) were of African origin, it was easier for us to observe that patients from around Buxton were much more likely to have a special cause of their hypertension. This is important, because the specific treatment for that condition is different.

It has been known for many years that African Americans on average have lower plasma renin levels. We have observed in our clinic that individuals from Africa, and individuals with African ancestors, are at least ten times more likely to have high blood pressure with low renin levels due to enlargement (hyperplasia) of the adrenal cortex. A recent study showed that another cause of low renin and high blood pressure accounted for 5 percent of hypertension in black persons (32): an abnormality of the kidney tubules that causes salt and water retention without heightened aldosterone. This condition, a variant of Liddle's syndrome, leads to low levels of both renin and aldosterone and is specifically treated with amiloride, one of the potassium-sparing diuretics.

The first patient in our clinic who required surgery for enlargement of the adrenal glands was a clergyman from Africa attending a seminary in our city. About a year after his surgery, he told me he was going back to Africa. Because we had taken out most of his adrenal tissue, I wrote a long letter for him to take home, explaining that he might need adrenal hormone replacement to prevent depletion of salt and water in the hot climate to which he was returning.

That experience made me wonder if having special ability to retain salt and water had a selective advantage in survival in hot countries. Subsequently, Dr. Clarence Grim of Los Angeles published a theory that having powerful adrenal glands might have conferred an advantage for survival of the Atlantic crossing in the conditions of terrible heat and privation between decks in slave ships (33).

Our experience is that individuals of African origin are more than ten times as likely to require surgery for enlargement of the adrenal cortex. This is a huge disproportion, and the recent report of the Liddle's syndrome variant accounting for 5 percent of hypertension in blacks suggests that stimulated plasma renin testing is particularly important for management of difficult hypertension among African Americans.

High blood pressure due to excess production of aldosterone is usually due to enlargement of both adrenal glands, often with multiple nodules, so it is called *nodular hyperplasia*. Many doctors think the problem is usually the result of a benign tumor of the adrenal gland (called *Conn's syndrome*, or *adrenal adenoma*), and many doctors believe the condition is curable with surgery. A minute fraction of individuals with primary hyperaldosteronism (that is, an enlargement of the adrenal cortex that causes overproduction of the adrenal gland hormone aldosterone) may be curable, but we found in the early 1980s that the problem is seldom, if ever, in only one adrenal gland. With Al Dreidger, we did nuclear medicine scans of one hundred individuals with abnormally low stimulated plasma renin levels (below 1 ng/ml/hr). Not a single case had only one adrenal gland involved; all were bilateral. Based on this experience, I believe that most people with primary hyperaldosteronism can manage it with medication, and that surgery should be reserved for those who cannot. The correct diagnosis points to the right medication, so less than 5 percent of my patients with primary hyperaldosteronism have required surgery.

Table 8.1 shows how measuring renin and aldosterone leads to the right primary treatment for individuals with resistant hypertension. Those with a low renin and high aldosterone have primary hyperaldosteronism, so the primary treatment is with drugs that block the effect of aldosterone on the kidney: spironolactone or eplerenone. (Amiloride can be used for men, where eplerenone is not available; men get breast enlargement from spironolactone.) Those with low renin and low aldosterone have salt and water retention due

Table 8.1 Rational Management of Resistant Hypertension

	Primary hyperaldosteronism	Liddle's syndrome	Renal or renovascular
Renin	Low	Low	High
Aldosterone	High	Low	High
Primary treatment	Spironolactone or eplerenone* (rarely surgery)	Amiloride	Angiotensin receptor antagonist (rarely surgery)

* Amiloride in high doses may be used where eplerenone is not available.

to an abnormality of the renal tubules (Liddle's syndrome and variants of it), and the primary treatment is amiloride. Those with high renin and high aldosterone have secondary hyperaldosteronism; their blood pressure and high levels of aldosterone are driven by kidney hormones, so they need kidney tests, and the primary treatment is with angiotensin receptor blockers.

The Bottom Line

If your blood pressure is difficult to control, or if you are having trouble with potassium depletion, and particularly if you have African ancestors, having your plasma renin and aldosterone measured after a dose of diuretic will be very helpful in pinpointing the cause of your hypertension and thus choosing the best treatment for you.

9
Adverse Drug Effects and How to Avoid Them

People deserve to receive good information about drugs they take and their possible serious adverse effects. Unfortunately, the information provided in most package inserts and handouts by pharmacists is worse than useless. The reason? The manufacturer is required to list every symptom ever experienced by anyone who has taken a drug. Therefore the lists tend to include all symptoms known to humankind, whether the reported symptoms were in fact caused by the drug, a flu, cancer, a hangover, or some other problem. All the lists thus tend to be similar and to include, for example, fatigue, nausea, dizziness, headache, vomiting, constipation, and diarrhea. (Does it make sense for such a list to include both diarrhea and constipation?) Seldom do we receive a list that would help us figure out whether a symptom is likely to be caused by the drug. Such a list would need to report the frequency of each symptom in individuals taking an inactive placebo (sugar pills) versus those taking the active drug.

The result of receiving such poor information is that if you experience a symptom and then find it on the list, you may stop the drug because the list seems to indicate a causal relationship, which is more often than not fallacious.

Just because you took the drug before the symptom showed up doesn't prove the drug caused the symptom. There may be other causes, such as a flu, a food allergy, or another coincidental cause. I believe this all-inclusive listing of possible side effects by drug manufacturers is responsible for a high and growing proportion of cases in which people who need safe and effective drugs inappropriately stop taking them. This syndrome probably contributes greatly to the poor control of blood pressure in North America: only about 25 percent of people with hypertension have it well controlled.

When considering whether to stop taking a drug, we need to balance the risk of taking it against the risk of stopping it. For example, if you have coronary artery disease or narrowing of a carotid artery, a cholesterol medication will reduce your risk of heart attack or death by 40 percent in six years. The risk of a serious adverse effect from the drug is about one in a thousand, so the balance is strongly in favor of staying on the medication unless there is strong evidence that the medication is causing the symptoms.

What we really need is a list of the symptoms that occur more often with the active drug than with a placebo, along with a focus on the important adverse effects of each drug. This chapter represents an effort to provide such information.

Calcium Channel Blockers (CCBs)

As we have seen, calcium-channel antagonists, or calcium-channel blockers, dilate arteries by interfering with the channels that permit calcium to enter cells. The significant differences in their adverse effects are summarized in Table 9.1.

If you are having trouble with constipation or shortness of breath (or other symptoms of heart failure—ask your doctor), changing from verapamil or diltiazem to another type of drug, or changing to a dihydropyridine (the largest class of CCBs) such as nifedipine, felodipine, or amlodipine should help.

If your problem is a slow heart rate from diltiazem, changing to a dihydropyridine or another class of drug should help; if it doesn't, check out whether you need a pacemaker. If you are on both dil-

Table 9.1. Adverse Effects of Calcium Channel Blockers

Drug Class	Main Adverse Effects
Verapamil	Constipation, aggravaion of congestive heart failure
Diltiazem	Slow heartbeat (bradycardia)
Dihydropyridines (nifedipine, felodipine, amlodipine)	Ankle swelling, fast heartbeat (tachycardia), headache

tiazem and a beta-blocker, the dose of beta-blocker may also need reducing.

If you're having a lot of angina on a dihydropyridine such as felodipine, adding a beta-blocker (or switching to diltiazem if you can't take a beta-blocker) should help. If it doesn't help, you should find out whether you need angioplasty or bypass surgery, and you should also be making sure that all the risk factors are optimally controlled. (Quitting smoking is the *most* important.)

If your problem is ankle swelling, flushing, or headache, switching from nifedipine or felodipine to amlodipine or another class of drug should help. Diltiazem and verapamil are not very strong and are extremely expensive, so I wouldn't usually advise using them for treating high blood pressure: the main reason to use them, in my opinion, is that verapamil is good for heart-rhythm disturbances such as atrial fibrillation, and diltiazem is good for angina (chest pain brought on by exertion, due to narrowing of the coronary arteries).

Beta-Adrenergic Blockers (Beta-Blockers)

With beta-blockers, the issue is the different ways individual bodies handle the drugs (pharmacokinetics) and the ways the drugs interact with adrenaline receptors (pharmacodynamics). Concerns in the ways bodies handle beta-blockers include how the drugs metabolize, how long the drug action lasts, how the drugs are absorbed into various body tissues, and how tightly the drug binds to receptors.

Metabolism

When food and drugs are absorbed into the bloodstream, the blood from the gut goes first to the liver to be detoxified before the heart pumps it around the body. Some drugs undergo extensive metabolism during absorption, either in the gut wall (see the section in Chapter 10 on effects of grapefruit juice on drug metabolism) or in the liver.

PROPRANOLOL AND METOPROLOL

Propranolol undergoes extensive metabolism during its first pass through the liver (first-pass metabolism); about 70 percent of an oral dose is broken down in the liver and never makes it to the rest of the body. There are huge differences among individuals in the extent to which the drug is metabolized. Both propranolol and metoprolol have a twenty-fold range in the blood levels achieved with a given dose. (That is, the same dose given to different people can lead to blood levels that range from five to one hundred units.)

This means that for some people, these two drugs can be expensive and may not work well, because the doctor is reluctant to prescribe a high enough dose. If you are one of these people, your hypertension will be much better controlled, at a much lower cost, with a beta-blocker that is excreted by the kidney or metabolized in a different way.

NADOLOL AND ATENOLOL

The two beta-blockers that are excreted by the kidney, nadolol and atenolol, create a special problem for the elderly and for people with impaired kidney function. They can build up in the bloodstream, causing relatively slow heart action (bradycardia), and aggravate heart failure, which in turn aggravates the kidney function, and a vicious circle can ensue. If you are on atenolol or nadolol and your heart rate has been getting slower and slower over months or years, ask your doctor to consider switching you to a beta-blocker that is not excreted by the kidney, but metabolized by the liver.

Duration of Drug Action

It is unnecessarily inconvenient to have to take pills more than once a day, but for reasons I do not understand, many doctors (especially cardiologists) prescribe metoprolol twice a day—often a half tablet twice a day, which is even more inconvenient.

The best and most convenient beta-blocker is pindolol, for several reasons. It has the most potent ISA, so it does not cause the adverse effects due to blockade of beta-2 receptors. (ISA, or intrinsic sympathomimetic activity, as discussed earlier, describes the action of drugs that block beta-1 receptors and stimulate beta-2 receptors.) Pindolol is also the best beta-blocker for people with diabetes, high cholesterol, or blocked arteries in the legs; as we will see, it is less likely to aggravate cholesterol and diabetes, and less likely to cause fatigue. It binds tightly to receptors, so it is long acting and can be taken only once daily. Finally, if doses are missed either by accident or through illness, it is the least likely to cause rebound hypertension. (When beta-blockers are suddenly stopped, the body reacts with a rise in heart rate and blood pressure that can be very severe; the pressures may be much higher than they ever were before treatment. This is called *rebound hypertension.* The same thing happens with clonidine.) The downside of pindolol is that a small proportion of people (about 5 percent) experience vivid dreams, tremor, or anxiety because of the drug's greater penetration into the brain, as described next.

Distribution into Body Tissues

The beta-blockers penetrate brain tissue to markedly varied extents because of marked differences in how well they dissolve in fat. Table 9.2 shows the ratios between levels of beta-blockers in the brain (central nervous system or CNS) and in blood plasma for a number of beta-blockers.

These differences in distribution, combined with the differences in the kind of receptors that are blocked and stimulated, explain why pindolol, with its extreme penetration into brain tissue, is the most likely beta-blocker to cause anxiety, tremors, and vivid dreams, and why propranolol, which is also concentrated in the brain, is the most likely to cause subjective tiredness and hallucinations.

If your problem is vivid dreams, tremor, or anxiety with pindolol,

Table 9.2 Brain Penetration of Beta-Blockers

Drug	CNS:Plasma Ratio
Pindolol	50:1
Propranolol	27:1
Metoprolol	3:1
Atenolol	1:3
Nadolol	1:4
Timolol	1:8

switching to acebutolol should avoid those problems while preserving most of the benefits of pindolol. Unfortunately, acebutolol should in most cases be taken twice a day.

Fatigue is a tricky problem. It can take at least two forms: subjective tiredness (feeling like you need a nap when you should be well rested), and fatigability (your legs turn to cement when you climb stairs).

If you are experiencing subjective tiredness with propranolol or metoprolol, changing to pindolol or atenolol should help. (The reason I suggest pindolol even though it gets readily into the brain is that it actually stimulates beta-2 receptors; that's why, in large doses, it causes anxiety and vivid dreams in about 5 percent of people. We will see the benefits of stimulating beta-2 receptors later.)

Fatigability can be due either to an excessive dose of beta-blocker that prevents the heart from speeding up to supply more blood to your muscles, or to differences in muscle blood flow or metabolism. If the problem is a low heart rate that won't go up with mild exercise like going up and down a couple of steps a few times, the problem is excessive beta-1 blockade, and reducing the dose is likely to work.

If the problem is reduced exercise capacity because of reduced muscle blood flow and metabolism (because of beta-2 blockade), then switching to pindolol or another class of drugs should help.

Receptor Binding

A special problem with beta-blockers (and with clonidine, a drug that is seldom used because this problem is so severe) is rebound hypertension if you miss even a couple of doses. This can happen when you forget to take the medication, when you can't keep it down because of a flu or other cause of vomiting, or when the drug is stopped for a reason such as surgery. This problem can be quite severe: I've seen two people whose usually controlled blood pressure bounced up to 240/140 after missing single doses of beta-blocker or clonidine. The first had his medication held for surgery, the other because of a burn that affected his mouth.

My friend Dr. Bob Rangno has shown that there is less rebound hypertension with pindolol, which in addition to its beta-2 stimulating activity has tighter binding to receptors; this means its effect takes a long time to wear off, and people are less likely to have problems with rebound (34).

Interaction with Receptors

Important considerations in how beta-blockers interact with the various receptors include selective blockade of beta-1 receptors (receptors that speed up the heart and cause it to beat harder) and stimulation of beta-2 receptors (those that cause dilation of the large air tubes in the lung and of the arteries that go to muscles).

Nonselective drugs such as propranolol, nadolol, and timolol are more likely to cause adverse effects due to beta-2 blockade.

Drugs that stimulate beta-2 receptors will have a different profile again: pindolol, a relatively potent beta-2 stimulator, has beneficial effects on cholesterol, may benefit diabetes, and is least likely to cause problems with cold extremities; fingers that get painful and turn red, white, and blue in the cold (Raynaud's phenomenon); and asthma.

Angiotensin-Converting Enzyme (ACE) Inhibitors

Any ACE inhibitor will cause a cough in about 8 percent of people, and swelling of the face and tongue (angioedema) in about one in one thousand. One can avoid these adverse effects by switching to angiotensin blockers, which have benefits similar to those of ACE inhibitors.

The first dose of any ACE inhibitor or angiotensin blocker can cause a severe drop in blood pressure, particularly in people taking diuretics. They can also cause acute kidney failure in people that have severe narrowing of both kidney arteries. This problem is rare; I have seen it only twenty times in more than four hundred patients with blockage of the kidney arteries, among the more than sixteen thousand patients I have seen. It is very unlikely to happen unless you have *very* severe high blood pressure, or heart failure. It is also reversible when the drug is stopped, in almost all cases.

Among ACE inhibitors, the main difference is due to the presence of a sulfhydryl group in captopril, which is responsible for the loss of taste and a characteristic generalized rash that looks like

Table 9.3 Pharmacodynamic Differences among Beta-Blockers

Receptor Type	Effects of Blockade	Adverse Effects
Beta 1	Reduced heart rate	Bradycardia
	Reduced contractility	Congestive failure
Beta 2	Vasoconstriction	Cold extremities, reduced muscle blood flow, Raynaud's phenomenon
	Bronchoconstriction	Aggravation of asthma
	Reduced insulin release	Aggravation of Type II diabetes
	Reduced gluconeogenesis	Aggravation of hypoglycemia by insulin
	Reduced fat metabolism	Aggravation of hyperlipidemia

measles. Both of these problems will disappear if you switch to another ACE inhibitor or to an angiotensin blocker.

Another difference that is occasionally important is in the duration of action. Captopril is very short acting and must be taken two or three times per day to achieve desired effects in all but the least severe cases. Lisinopril, quinapril, and some of the other ACE inhibitors are long acting enough to work well when taken once a day.

Captopril is also the most expensive of the ACE inhibitors (for an equivalent effect). Given its problems with rash, loss of taste, short duration of action, and high cost, I never prescribe it. The main place for it in my opinion is in starting therapy in persons with heart failure, who may require very small doses of ACE inhibitor at first to avoid a blood-pressure crash. (It is quite likely that the crash in blood pressure in these individuals is due to unrecognized narrowing of the kidney arteries: one study in the *Lancet* showed that more than 30 percent of individuals with heart failure have a kidney artery narrowing that aggravates the heart failure but goes unrecognized because the heart is so weak that it cannot maintain the characteristic high blood pressure usually associated with kidney artery narrowing.) (35)

Diuretics

Potassium Depletion

People taking long-term diuretic therapy—that is, medication to rid their body of salt and water—often experience adverse effects related to depletion of a number of ions. Often the rubric *hypokalemia* (low blood level of potassium) is used to characterize the problem. Most doctors think that the condition will be diagnosed by measuring serum potassium and resolved with potassium supplements. In most cases these assumptions are incorrect.

The problem is not a low level of potassium in the blood, it is potassium depletion in the cells throughout the body, including muscles, heart, brain, and elsewhere. Potassium supplements do not restore intracellular potassium unless magnesium is taken at the same time. The problem is not trivial: maintaining adequate intracellular potassium helps prevent toxicity of digoxin (a heart medication that can cause serious problems if the blood level is too high, or the potassium level in the cells is too low) and minimizes the adverse effects of diuretics on diabetes and cholesterol.

Taking diuretics causes the body to react by turning on hormone systems designed to retain salt and water. As discussed earlier, the kidney makes more of an enzyme called renin, which activates angiotensin I. Angiotensin I is converted to its active form, angiotensin II, by an enzyme called angiotensin-converting enzyme (ACE). Angiotensin II is a powerful hormone that constricts arteries, promotes thickening of the arteries and the heart, and also stimulates the adrenal gland to produce aldosterone.

Aldosterone causes the kidney to retain sodium and excrete potassium and other ions (see Figure 9.1); when potassium is eventually depleted, there is excretion of hydrogen ions, leading to an alkaline state in the blood (alkalosis).

For individuals with normal serum potassium levels and with digoxin levels in the therapeutic range, digoxin toxicity can be predicted by alkaline urine, which is an indicator of intracellular potassium depletion. Most individuals with potassium depletion have a normal serum potassium (36). Thus, measuring serum potassium does not diagnose the problem; indeed, it is very common (even usual) for persons with significant potassium depletion to have a normal serum potassium. At present, the best test we have is how you feel. If you are taking a diuretic and feel tired, achy, have cramps in your extremities, are impotent, and feel faint when you stand up, the chances are very good that you have depleted potassium. Usually when there is potassium depletion, there is also depletion of magnesium, zinc, selenium, rubidium, and other ions.

Although it is not certain which ion depletion causes impotence, we know that zinc depletion causes fatigue, nausea, impaired wound healing, and hair loss. Magnesium is a cofactor for an enzyme that regulates movement of sodium and potassium across cell membranes such as the kidney tubules, and muscle cells. For that reason, for people with depleted magnesium and potassium, even intravenous administration of potassium does not correct intracellular potassium depletion unless magnesium is taken at the same time. The upshot of all this is that it is better to prevent depletion of potassium and magnesium, since taking potassium alone doesn't work, and magnesium is hard to take by mouth (it often causes diarrhea).

Since potassium-sparing diuretics are also magnesium sparing, they prevent both magnesium and potassium depletion and are more effective at restoring intracellular ions.

Similarly, drugs that reduce production of aldosterone by the adrenal gland also are magnesium and potassium sparing. Drugs that block activation of angiotensin by blocking angiotensin-converting enzyme (ACE inhibitors such as captopril, enalapril, lisinopril, or any drug with a proper name ending in -*pril*), or by blocking angiotensin II at its receptor (losartan, irbesartan, candesartan, or other drugs ending in -*sartan*), will reduce urinary losses of potassium, magnesium, and probably the other ions that are depleted by diuretics. (These examples show why it is better to use generic names than trade names: the generic names tell you what kind of drug they are.)

Salt Intake

Because potassium loss from the kidney is driven by exchange of potassium for sodium as regulated by aldosterone, salt intake is an important concern. The more salt you eat, the more potassium you lose. As Figure 9.1 illustrates, every sodium ion reabsorbed from the renal tubule leads to excretion of a potassium ion; high sodium intake aggravates potassium losses, and when potassium is depleted, potassium ions are exchanged for hydrogen ions, leading to acid urine with alkaline blood.

To minimize potassium losses, then, one can reduce salt intake; use angiotensin-receptor blockers (ARBs) to prevent angiotensin II from causing the adrenal cortex to release aldosterone; or block

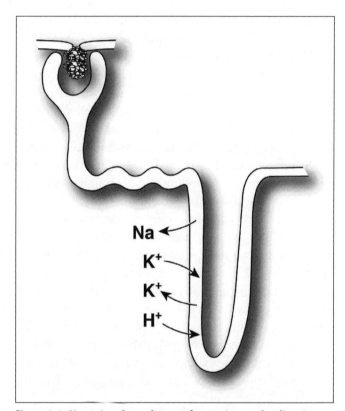

Figure 9.1 Upsetting the exchange of potassium and sodium ions in the kidney tubules can cause potassium depletion in the cells throughout the body. Every sodium ion (NA) reabsorbed from the renal tubule leads to excretion of a potassium ion (K); high sodium intake aggravates potassium losses, and when potassium is depleted, potassium ions are exchanged for hydrogen ions (H), leading to acid urine with alkaline blood.

the effect of aldosterone on the kidney tubule by using potassium/magnesium-sparing diuretics.

Potassium Supplements

For the vast majority of people who take diuretics, routine potassium supplements are not necessary.

For people with problems, particularly those who exhibit symptoms of potassium/magnesium depletion or who show hypokalemia on their laboratory tests, a simple solution usually resolves the issue, as we will see. In my Hypertension Clinic, which in its first ten years enrolled more than four thousand people with difficult hypertension, (including two hundred with adrenocortical hypertension and more than four hundred with renovascular hypertension), the approach described in the next section was successful in the vast majority. We have only two patients who require long-term potassium supplementation; both appear to have rare renal tubular problems.

Available potassium supplements leave much to be desired. Since the normal daily intake of potassium in the diet is 80–100 mEq/day, a tablet containing only 8 mEq does not contribute much to potassium balance. In addition to cost, these supplements may have adverse effects, including gastrointestinal (GI) erosions and GI bleeding.

Larger doses of potassium supplements in liquid form are less likely to cause gastric irritation, but their taste is disagreeable.

An Approach to Managing Potassium/Magnesium Depletion

Potassium depletion can usually be managed by a combination of reducing your salt intake, reducing the dose of diuretic, and using either potassium/magnesium-sparing diuretics or drugs that prevent excess aldosterone production such as angiotensin receptor blockers.

RESTRICTING SALT

Reducing your sodium intake is much easier than you may think; see "How to Reduce Salt Intake" in Chapter 8.

REDUCING THE DOSE OF DIURETIC

For most individuals, particularly the elderly, a daily dose of 12.5 mg hydrochlorothiazide (HCTZ, the commonest and cheapest drug for treating high blood pressure) is enough; if your pressure is not controlled by that dose, it is better to add another drug than to increase it. It is widely understood now that doses above 12.5 mg daily mainly achieve increased adverse effects.

In persons with heart failure, spironolactone or amiloride, or ACE inhibitors or ARBs, will minimize requirements for other diuretics. With all these drugs, but particularly amiloride and spironolactone, it is important to have blood tests to guard against high potassium levels. With spironolactone it is also necessary to guard against accumulation of digoxin, because spironolactone reduces the excretion of digoxin by the kidney.

USING POTASSIUM/MAGNESIUM-SPARING DIURETICS

Among diuretics that do not deplete the body's potassium and magnesium, amiloride is generally preferred for men, because men who take spironolactone often have sore nipples and sometimes breast enlargement. This does not appear to be a problem with eplerenone, a new aldosterone antagonist. I would also avoid triamterene, because half the people who take it develop an abnormality in the urine (triamterene casts) (37), and it is implicated in kidney inflammation (interstitial nephritis) and kidney stones.

The key to using these drugs is to get the proportion right with respect to the dose of other diuretics. Often people with severe potassium depletion (for instance, with hypertension from enlargement of the adrenal glands, or with tremendously increased aldosterone levels secondary to high renin levels from renal artery stenosis) will be better off with only a potassium-sparing diuretic in large doses. (As we have seen, overproduction of aldosterone because of high levels of renin and angiotensin is called *secondary hyperaldosteronism*.)

If a small dose of one of the thiazide family of diuretics is required, a common ratio might be HCTZ 12.5 mg to amiloride 10–20 mg, or spironolactone 100 mg. For people with secondary hyperaldosteronism (the tip-off is a high stimulated renin level), angiotensin receptor blockers are more effective.

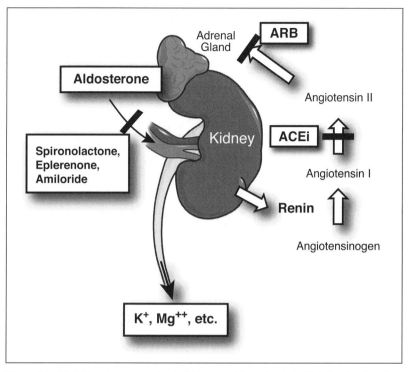

Figure 9.2   High blood pressure due to kidney problems leads to high levels of renin, which produce high levels of angiotensin II; these are best blocked by angiotensin-receptor blockers (ARBs).

USING ANGIOTENSIN RECEPTOR BLOCKERS (ARBS)

When you take diuretics, your body turns on renin, a kidney enzyme intended to preserve salt and water, and triggers a cycle that produces angiotensin II, a potent vasoconstrictor that leads the adrenal cortex to release aldosterone, a hormone that as we have seen causes the kidney to retain salt and water and to excrete potassium and magnesium (Figure 9.2).

Blocking the effect of high renin—that is, potassium and magnesium depletion—by blocking the effect of angiotensin II with angiotensin receptor blockers (ARBs) will prevent secondary hyperaldosteronism.

This may be the best approach for people who have either congestive heart failure or secondary hyperaldosteronism from renal artery stenosis or other high-renin states. ACE inhibitors, soon after they are started, also block formation of angiotensin II, but this effect wears off after a few weeks because there are other pathways for the formation of angiotensin II. It is very important to understand that if potassium-sparing diuretics and ARBs or ACE inhibitors are used together, there is a real risk of seriously increased levels of potassium in the blood (hyperkalemia).

For primary hyperaldosteronism the specific treatment is blockers of aldosterone such as spironolactone and eplerenone; amiloride can also be used and is the specific treatment for hypertension due to abnormalities of the renal tubule such as Liddle's syndrome.

The Bottom Line

In summary, the problem is not low levels of potassium in the blood (hypokalemia) but potassium/magnesium depletion; potassium supplements do not solve the problem because magnesium is required to restore intracellular potassium. A recommended approach is to:

- reduce salt intake toward 2–3 grams per day
- reduce the dose of diuretic
- use potassium/magnesium-sparing diuretics to prevent losses, *or*
- use angiotensin blockers to reduce secondary hyperaldosteronism and thus prevent depletion of potassium and magnesium.

The best approach to prevention of potassium depletion is different for people with high plasma renin as opposed to low plasma renin, as we have seen.

Statins

Muscle Problems

Statins are drugs that inhibit cholesterol synthesis in the liver by inhibiting an enzyme, HMG-CoA reductase. Their most common side effect is aching and cramps in the muscles, caused by depletion

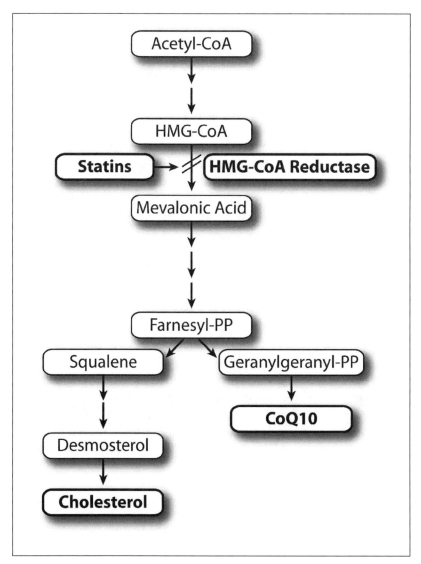

Figure 9.3   Statins lower levels not only of cholesterol in the liver by inhibiting the enzyme HMG-CoA reductase but also of all the metabolites along the metabolic pathway, including one that helps makes CoQ10, whose depletion can cause muscle cramps and aching.

of ubiquinone, also called co-enzyme Q10 (CoQ10). This happens because inhibiting the liver enzyme HMG-CoA reductase lowers not only cholesterol levels but also the levels of all the metabolites along the pathway, including one that is used to make CoQ10 (see Figure 9.3). The mitochondria (the metabolic engines of the cells) in the muscles need CoQ10 to work properly, so its depletion can cause muscle cramps and aching.

There is now some evidence from Dr. Rene Vladutiu and her colleagues in Buffalo, New York, that people who develop muscle problems with statins have a genetic predisposition because of metabolic abnormalities that affect the function of the mitochondria (38). This problem, which occurs in about 5–10 percent of people, can be managed by taking supplements of CoQ10. Dr. Patricia Kelly and her colleagues of Stoney Brook, New York, have shown that supplements of CoQ10 reduce muscle pain from statins (39); I have observed the same effect in my clinic, and I am also conducting a study on this issue. (In my experience about 60–120 mg of CoQ10 twice a day is enough for most people.)

Another approach is to reduce the dose of statin and add ezetimibe, a drug that lowers cholesterol by blocking its absorption in the lining of the intestine. Ezetimibe doesn't affect the muscles, but it helps the statin work eight times better, so a much lower dose of statin will still be effective. New drugs that selectively block the formation of squalene so they don't affect CoQ10 are in development (see Figure 9.3).

10

Vitamins, Homocysteine, and Grapefruit Juice

Besides knowing about drugs, it is also important to know about some natural products—vitamins and foods—that affect cardiovascular health or the metabolism of drugs.

Vitamins

A number of chemicals, including vitamins, that we obtain largely through our diet have important functions as cofactors, or partners, in chemical reactions in the body.

Vitamins are properly used mainly as supplements to treat deficits. A deficit of vitamin B_{12}, for example, can result from various causes with disparate results. "Pernicious anemia" is a condition in which vitamin B_{12} is not properly absorbed because the stomach does not produce a factor required for its absorption in the distal intestine. Individuals who lack this factor can develop anemia, because we need vitamin B_{12} to make new red blood cells; they can also develop a problem with the spinal cord and peripheral nerves that results in numbness and tingling of the extremities and, if untreated, in paralysis and dementia.

Another cause of vitamin B_{12} depletion is long-term use of drugs that suppress the production of acid by the stomach, such as omeprazole. We need gastric acid to strip vitamin B_{12} off food so we can absorb it; because crystalline vitamin B_{12} can be absorbed from tablets without acid, it will be effective. Individuals taking omeprazole or related drugs for longer than a few months should probably take a B_{12} supplement.

For the most part, a balanced diet provides sufficient amounts of vitamins, and few individuals have deficits. Exceptions exist, though, particularly for vitamin B_{12} and folic acid.

Vegetarians and the elderly are often deficient in B_{12}. Because the main dietary source of B_{12} is meat, most vegetarians do not consume enough of the vitamin, so they should take a B_{12} supplement. Regarding the elderly, the Framingham Heart Study, a long-term study of cardiovascular risk factors that has been going on for about thirty years in Framingham, Massachusetts, found that a surprisingly high proportion of elderly persons had low levels of folic acid or vitamin B_{12}. It is now apparent that about 15–20 percent of the elderly have B_{12} deficiency (40). This is often (usually) missed because many doctors do not understand the meaning of the word *normal* as it applies to blood levels. The "normal curve," or bell-shaped curve, is a statistical definition that includes the 95 percent of the population within two standard deviations from the average level of whatever is being measured, such as serum B_{12}. By definition, it excludes only the top 2.5 percent and the bottom 2.5 percent of the population. However, when adequate levels of vitamin B_{12} are defined by the metabolic effect of B_{12} (assessed by measuring methylmalonic acid), it turns out that 20 percent of people over age sixty-five (40)—and in my clinic, 30 percent of people over age seventy—have inadequate levels of B_{12}. This means that the "normal" range includes 17.5 percent of people above age sixty-five with inadequate B_{12} levels, and 27.5 percent above age seventy.

Folic acid is particularly important for the development of the nervous system in the fetus. A typical North American diet, which can be characterized as tasty meat and boring vegetables, may not provide enough folic acid for pregnant women; it is now apparent that folic acid fortification of cereal-grain products (mandated in the United States since 1998) has reduced by half abnormalities of the brain and spinal cord that lead to spina bifida and related abnormalities (neural tube defects).

Folic Acid and Vitamins: Treatment for High Homocysteine

High Blood Levels of Homocysteine

As we have learned, homocysteine is an amino acid (a building block of protein) produced in the body that may increase blood clotting and irritate blood vessels, leading to blockages in the arteries. High blood levels of this substance were first identified as a problem in young people with seizures, premature strokes, abnormalities of the lens of the eye, and developmental problems: all have very high blood levels of homocysteine and related compounds and excrete homocystine (which is like two homocysteine molecules attached) in the urine. This original form (called *homocystinuria* because homocystine was excreted in the urine) is due to an inherited deficiency in the enzyme that converts homocysteine to another amino acid, cystathionine. To do its work, that enzyme needs vitamin B_6, also called *pyridoxine*, as a cofactor.

I believe that in part because the original cause was rare, this condition has been unduly neglected. It is actually quite common:, high blood levels of total homocysteine (tHcy, which means the total of three variants of homocysteine in the blood) affect about 20 percent of North Americans, and about half of individuals who have artery problems at a young age and who don't have the traditional risk factors.

Artery Damage from Homocysteine

It appears that homocysteine creates problems by producing free radicals such as hydrogen peroxide and by damaging the inner lining of the artery (the endothelium). Free radicals are chemically active compounds that, among other negative reactions, oxidize LDL cholesterol; homocysteine also consumes nitric oxide, the protective substance produced by the artery wall. High blood levels of homocysteine therefore increase the activation of platelets and blood clotting, cause constriction of the arteries, and cause proliferation of smooth muscle cells in the artery wall. This proliferation of smooth muscle cells is atherosclerosis, blockage in the arteries.

Approaches to Treatment

The reason high blood levels of homocysteine are so important is that the condition is so easily treated. Folic acid 2.5 mg. daily will normalize blood levels of homocysteine in about half the cases; a combination of folic acid 1mg, vitamin B_6 10 mg, and vitamin B_{12} 1000 mcg (= 1 mg) will normalize levels in more than 95 percent of cases. We have recently learned that the dose of B_{12} needs to be higher than we used to think. In the elderly, 1000 mcg per day is necessary for some people, and a few need an even higher dose to ensure sufficient absorption. An even better approach is a 1200 mcg slow-release tablet. I recommend having the B_{12} level checked about a month after starting B_{12}, to make sure the blood level is above 300 pmol/L.

In some cases it is necessary to add a fourth supplement called betaine, and vitamins are not as effective for individuals with kidney failure (for them we are now working on new therapies). Overnight daily dialysis is more effective at lowering homocysteine than routine dialysis three times a week, and sulfur-containing compounds called *thiols* may be useful.

A Swiss study of individuals who had undergone coronary angioplasty showed that vitamin therapy with folate, B_6, and B_{12} reduced the occurrence of a reconstriction of the coronary arteries (restenosis) and also reduced combined events (heart attack, death, and surgery or stenting to open the coronary arteries) (41, 42). In the recent NORVIT and HOPE-TOO studies, and in another study that showed negative results (43), I believe the researchers used too low a dose of B_{12}. A large North American study that I participated in, the Vitamin Intervention for Stroke Prevention (VISP) trial (44), failed to show a benefit for vitamin therapy in stroke patients, but that null result can be explained by several factors: folic acid fortification of the North American grain supply coincided with the initiation of the study, thus negating the benefit of the folic acid in the study treatment and we also treated anyone in the study who had deficiency of B_{12} with injections of vitamin B_{12}, so we ended up showing, essentially, that vitamin B_6 by itself does not prevent recurrent stroke. When we analyzed the subgroup of patients who were more likely to respond (after excluding those who received nonstudy supplements and injections of B_{12}, and those with kidney failure), the vitamin therapy was effective in preventing stroke, death, and coronary events (45). A large study called the VITATOPS study is still under way, so there are more discoveries to come.

If you are a woman of child-bearing age, you should have your plasma homocysteine measured: women with high levels are much more likely to have babies with neural tube defects such as spina bifida, and they need higher than usual doses of vitamins to reduce that risk. Since the damage to the baby occurs in the first month of pregnancy, women with high homocysteine levels need to know about this condition before they are pregnant. If you think you may have this problem, you need your blood level checked before you treat it, so that if you do have high plasma homocysteine, everyone in your family can find out if they need vitamins. (If you have a high homocysteine level, you may have one of the genetic causes of elevated homocysteine; there are about ten such conditions.)

Vitamins and Antioxidants

Recently there has been a lot of interest in the idea that vitamin E, vitamin C, and beta carotene, which reduce oxidation, may be protective. An important rationale for such a possibility is that the harmful form of cholesterol is probably oxidized low-density lipoprotein (LDL) cholesterol, and antioxidant vitamins may reduce oxidation of LDL. Another issue is that at about age seventy, one experiences a marked increase in a number of markers of oxidation. The way antioxidants work can be understood by picturing how a sliced apple or banana exposed to the oxygen in air turns brown (the result of combining with the oxygen, that is, oxidation), but lemon juice, which contains vitamin C, delays the oxidation and discoloration.

VITAMIN E

One study from Cambridge showed a significant reduction in recurrent heart attacks in individuals given vitamin E after a heart attack. (Much has been made of the fact that the number of individuals who died in the course of the study was not reduced by the vitamin; however the study was not large enough to show an effect on mortality, and when larger studies are done we will have the answer to that part of the question.) A recent analysis of results from a number of studies showed that vitamin E taken on its own was harmful. This could be because vitamin E, when it accepts a free radical, itself becomes a free radical (the tocophyryl radical); it then needs vitamin C to come along and detoxify it. A Finnish study showed that combining vitamin E with 250 mg daily of slow-release vitamin C reduced the progression of artery thickening as measured by ultrasound (46).

However, in addition to the multistudy analysis, a substudy of the HOPE study found that vitamin E was associated with an excess of heart failure. Recently a large study funded by NIH, the Women's Health Initiative, showed that vitamin E reduced cardiovascular mortality but did not clearly reduce the number of heart attacks and strokes (47). Thus it seems that vitamin E by itself is not helpful and may be harmful. That vitamin E may be beneficial in combination with vitamin C is suggested by the Finnish study just described.

This raises the issue of combinations of vitamins. It is probably best to get our vitamins and antioxidants from food rather than from tablets. Vitamin C in orange juice or grapefruit juice, for example, brings along with it other potentially beneficial antioxidants and bioflavonoids: hesperitin in orange juice and naringin in grapefruit juice are related to genistein in soy beans. These have anticancer and cholesterol-lowering effects. The antioxidant lycopene is what gives the red color to tomatoes, watermelon, and strawberries; blueberries get their color and flavor from another brightly colored antioxidant. It is therefore a good idea to *eat fruits and vegetables of all colors,* to get a variety of antioxidants from our diet.

The Grapefruit Effect on Drug Metabolism

In 1990, my colleagues David Bailey, Claudio Munoz, and Malcolm Arnold and I discovered a surprising effect of grapefruit juice on drug metabolism (48). The discovery was a true example of serendipity: we set out to study the effect of alcohol on the metabolism and effects of a blood-pressure drug called felodipine, and we used grapefruit juice only because it masked the flavor of the alcohol better than orange juice did, so we could do a blinded study.

Because both felodipine and alcohol dilate blood vessels, we suspected there might be more flushing and faintness when felodipine was taken with alcohol; we saw no effects from alcohol on the metabolism of felodipine. To our surprise, however, the blood levels of felodipine were about three times higher than expected on both the alcohol and non-alcohol day. We excluded the obvious possibility that the manufacturer had given us a stronger tablet of felodipine, and then we tested the effect of taking felodipine with grapefruit juice versus with water, using Dr. Bailey as our subject. We didn't need to wait for the blood level results to come back from Sweden to see the effect: he turned red as a beet and had a very low blood pressure on the grapefruit-juice day. It turned out that his felodipine blood levels were six times higher on the day he took the drug with grapefruit juice!

That chance observation led to a series of studies that have shown that grapefruit juice inhibits the metabolism of a number of drugs. What these drugs have in common is that during absorption, a large proportion of the drug is metabolized by oxidation to form another chemical, in the wall of the intestine. This oxidation is performed by a specific form of the family of oxidative enzymes (Cytochrome P450) called CYP3A4. Drugs that are largely metabolized during oxidation are said to have low bioavailability, because a low proportion of the drug is available to the body. When the metabolism of these drugs in the intestinal wall is inhibited, a much larger proportion of the drug is absorbed unchanged, and the blood levels of the drug are much higher.

It turned out that felodipine had a bioavailability of only 15 percent, so its blood levels on average were tripled by grapefruit juice (43), and its effects on blood pressure and heart rate were doubled. It turns out also that within the family of drugs to which felodipine belongs (called the dihydropyridine calcium-channel antagonists), those drugs with high bioavailability such as amlodipine are not much affected by grapefruit juice; nifedipine, which is 60 percent bioavailable, has a 30 percent rise in blood levels when taken with grapefruit juice, and nisoldipine, which is 8 percent bioavailable, goes up on average fivefold, with a range of up to ninefold!

Interestingly, ordinary Florida orange juice had no such effect, though Seville orange juice and lime juice have some effect (though less powerful than those of grapefruit juice), and the search has been on for the active ingredients in grapefruit juice that cause this remarkable effect. So far it appears that a furanocoumarin derivative, bergamottin and related compounds, is responsible for the effect on drug oxidation, whereas naringin inhibits a different mechanism of drug handling; a drug pump called organic anion transport protein (OATP) also is affected by grapefruit. Drs. Bailey, George Dresser, Richard Kim, and others are still working on that.

Other drugs for which the grapefruit-juice effect is important include the transplant antirejection drug cyclosporine (a tripling of blood levels); the AIDS drug saquinovir (large effects); the sleeping pills midazolam and triazolam; and most importantly, the antihistamine terfenadine. Both terfenadine and the gut-motility drug cisapride can cause serious heart-rhythm disturbances when their metabolism is inhibited. A large part of why terfenadine and cisapride are no longer on the market is probably their interaction with grapefruit. The problem is that although your pharmacist will take a drug history before dispensing a new drug, a grocer seldom takes a drug history before dispensing grapefruit!

Other drugs affected importantly by grapefruit include the anticoagulant warfarin and the heart-rhythm drug propafenone in some individuals, and the cholesterol-lowering drugs lovastatin and simvastatin. Blood levels of both lovastatin and simvastatin can be increased fifteen-fold by a glass of grapefruit juice. Atorvastatin is also affected by grapefruit, although to a much lesser degree, but pravastatin and rosuvastatin are not. A simple rule of thumb is that if a drug should not be taken with erythromycin, ketoconazole or itraconazole, it should not be taken with grapefruit juice.

Two important issues have been widely misinterpreted: dose of grapefruit juice, and timing. It turns out that the effect of grapefruit juice increases with repeated dosing, that the effect persists for more than twenty-four hours, and that a single glass of normal strength grapefruit juice produces most of the effect observed in our original study, in which we used "double-strength" juice. Recommendations that the drug not be taken until four hours after drinking grapefruit juice, or that a small amount of juice is okay, are therefore mistaken. To be safe, you should not drink grapefruit juice if you are taking one of the affected drugs. Have orange juice instead, or change to a drug that is not affected.

A Guide to Healthy Meals
Gourmet Vegetable-Based Cooking

The Importance of Diet

Diet is much more important than most doctors think. I think that's because of a misplaced focus on the cholesterol level you wake up with (the fasting cholesterol level), which is not much affected by diet. The fasting cholesterol level is like a baseline, which shows what the artery lining has been exposed to overnight; however, for about eighteen hours of the day, what affects the artery lining is the fats from meals, on top of that baseline. So 75 percent of the day's exposure to cholesterol and harmful fat is determined by diet.

The Lyon Diet Heart Study (23) showed that a Mediterranean diet from Crete reduced heart attacks and death by 60 percent in four years, compared to the diet usually prescribed in North American coronary care units. This was recently confirmed in a study in India (24).

A Cretan Mediterranean diet is low in cholesterol and animal fat, high in beneficial oils such as olive and canola, and high in fruit, vegetables, and whole-grain fiber.

What You Should Aim For

- Never eat an egg yolk (use whites or substitutes such as Egg Beaters or Better than Eggs).
- Avoid trans fats and fried foods such as chips and fries.
- Keep your meat intake to two ounces per day, or one serving of animal flesh of any kind every other day—an animal is

anything with eyes, a face, or a mother; fish is better than chicken, which is better than beef.

- Use a nonhydrogenated canola margarine, preferably one that also contains olive oil.
- Instead of thinking of your meatless day as your punishment day, think of it as your gourmet cooking-class day. Have fun making vegetarian meals delicious. A positive attitude is what it takes to make a big change in lifelong habits.

Finding Alternatives

One of the key issues is finding alternatives for the "fat bombs" like potato chips, French fries, butter, ice cream, and sour cream (see "Calorie Bombs" in the chart). Think of your calories as hard-earned money that you have saved up. Don't blow them on things you don't really want, and think of really high-calorie foods as having too high a price tag.

For instance, try low-fat yogurt in place of sour cream for vegetable dips and baked potatoes. You can also make low-fat yogurt into a cheese spread by putting it in a coffee filter and draining out the water; this can replace cream cheese for bagels, and in lasagna and other dishes that call for cheese.

If you have diabetes, are overweight, or have a high triglyceride level, reducing sugar intake is important. The best sugar substitute, especially for cooking, is sucralose (Splenda) because it is closest to the texture of sugar and doesn't lose its flavor with heating. It can be used in baking, in making sorbet, and even in cocktails.

For sautéing, use a nonstick wok or pan, and instead of oil, use a nonstick spray such as Pam, or the President's Choice Virtuous Spray. A 1.5-second spray is seven calories of fat, compared to almost fifty in a teaspoon of oil!

Use popcorn instead of potato chips or nuts. Obviously, the popcorn should not be greasy, salty bags of popcorn, but kernels popped in the microwave or an air popper; a teaspoon of canola margarine is 50 calories, so try spices or other flavorings with your popcorn instead of a lot of margarine or butter. The baked potato should not be stuffed with butter and sour cream, but with some-

Calorie Bombs	Alternative
Peanuts (7 each)	Popcorn
Cashews (15 each)	Popcorn
Potato chips (10 each)	Popcorn
French fries (600)	Baked potato
Big store-bought muffin (450)	Low-fat muffin (200)
Cooking oil (50/teaspoon)	Non-stick spray, 1.5 seconds (7)
Ice cream, 2 scoops (400)	Sugarless sorbet (100)
Meat (400)	Baked potato, large (200)
Salad dressing (125/tbsp)	Low-fat (70)
Chili with meat, 8 oz (400)	Meatless chili (200)

thing like low-fat yogurt (stir in a bit of mustard powder and green onion or chives).

For the most part, sugarless sorbet would need to be homemade (with Splenda); there may be sugarless brands of sorbet available of which I am not aware.

Figuring Weight Loss

One pound of fat consists of 3,500 calories stored. That means that to lose a pound, you need to cut out 500 calories a day for a week; to lose 50 pounds you need to cut out 500 calories a day for 50 weeks; to keep it off you need to cut out 500 calories a day permanently. (To lose 20 pounds, you would need to cut out about 200 calories a day.)

One serving of anything fat-based, such as meat, cake, pie, ice cream, nuts, chips, or fries, is about 400 calories; a serving of starches or sugars, such as potatoes, pasta, rice, bread, juice, fruit, four crackers, half a bagel, or a can of pop, is 100 calories. If you stay away from cake, pie, ice cream (except on your birthday), nuts, chips, and fries; keep your meat intake to one serving every other day; and keep optional sugars and starches (meaning the ones not part of the main meal) to five or six a day, you will lose weight. The trick is finding alternatives you like.

Making Vegetable-Based Meals Delicious

Hints for Tasty, Interesting Stir-Fry Meals

- **The sauce:** Prepare this in advance and have it handy next to the stove. Any stir-fry dish can employ sauce to blend flavors and enhance the accompaniment of rice. The basic trick is to run hot tap water slowly into a cup with a fork-ful of cornstarch and quickly stir to produce a thin paste. (A heaping forkful is about the same as a tablespoon, but it stirs better.) Gradually add more water or wine (up to about three-quarters of a cup) and a teaspoon of Hoisin sauce or peanut butter, or a bit of hot sauce. Different sauces enhance different dishes; for instance, beef with green peppers, green onions, and snow peas goes well with peanut butter and hot sauce, whereas white wine plus a tablespoon of Hoisin sauce would enhance a vegetable stir-fry.

- **Preparation.** For ease of preparation, have all items chopped up ahead of time. Separate harder vegetables such as celery and carrots from softer ones such as mushrooms. I like to put them in small bowls ready to toss into the wok. Spray the nonstick wok with Pam or a similar spray, or heat a small amount of oil in the wok (canola oil is a good choice because it is high in monounsaturated fats and takes the heat better than olive oil). Add finely-chopped fresh ginger and/or garlic (or pre-chopped from a jar) for flavor. Cook the hard vegetables first (e.g., carrots, celery, cauliflower, broccoli) with a quick stir. Add a couple of tablespoons or so of water, put the lid on the wok, and steam them for about a minute. Take the lid off, add softer vegetables (such as zucchini, onions, mushrooms) and continue to stir until vegetables are almost cooked. Scoop out a well in the middle of the vegetables and pour in the cornstarch sauce. As it thickens, stir the vegetables until they are coated with sauce, then quickly remove from the wok into a large bowl. Serve immediately. Rice is a suitable accompaniment; brown rice is better because it is more slowly converted to sugar.

- **Wok maintenance:** To avoid rust on an iron wok, rinse it with hot water and scrub immediately after cooking, then pour a bit of oil in the bottom and wipe it evenly with a paper towel to coat the wok. Using a nonstick wok is helpful in reducing the requirements for oil; an electric wok may be helpful since it is more efficient than sitting a wok on top of an electric burner. If you have a gas stove, then a regular wok on top of a gas burner is probably the best choice. For an electric range you need a wok with a flat bottom. A wok with a long wooden handle is easier to use than one that has two small handles requiring two hands to lift, which leaves you no hand free for the spatula or scrub brush for quick rinses between dishes.

Microwaving Vegetables

A microwave oven is convenient for cooking vegetables. Add just a bit of water to any type of fresh or frozen vegetables and cook briefly to produce a crisp product. Preparation is easy and takes very little time. The microwave dish can often double as a serving dish. Any leftovers can go into the freezer in same dish, and be re-heated in the microwave the next day, and still remain surprisingly fresh.

Frozen Vegetables

In addition to variety, convenience, and freshness, another advantage of frozen over canned vegetables is that canned vegetables have a considerable amount of salt added to them, and you are trying to avoid salt.

Meatless Days

One hint that may help you in preparing more-balanced meals is to choose two or three days a week as meatless days. This will force you to find vegetable dishes with "star quality" and make it easier for you to include them in your menus on other days of the week.

Variety

Most households rotate about fifteen main meals through the kitchen. To make a substantial change, you will need to find about a dozen vegetable-based or pasta meals that you like and that are reasonable to prepare. Then you will need to change your grocery-shopping habits to be sure you replace the staple ingredients for those meals on a regular basis.

The whole secret to making a major change in your diet is a positive attitude: instead of thinking, "He's telling me I have to cut out everything I like!" make up your mind to have fun learning how to make healthy meals delicious.

When you go to a restaurant, use it as an opportunity to learn a new dish for your repertoire. Try a Chinese, Indian, or other restaurant that offers interesting vegetarian choices and ask the server to help you order a vegetarian meal; if you like the dishes, figure out how you can make them at home. Explore the cuisine of poor countries, where meat is a luxury.

Recipes

Because I was born and raised in Peru, I love spicy food. If some of these recipes are too spicy for you, cut back on the spices. If you don't like curry, leave out the curry powder, and call the dish chili or stew!

If you don't like these recipes, tinker with them until you do, or try others. Tolerably good is not good enough; if you don't like the result, you won't make it.

Legumes, such as beans, lentils, chickpeas, and nuts are important because legumes and grains together make up a complete protein. Grains and legumes are each missing some of the amino acids, but combining them gets you all of the essential amino acids; it is likely for that reason that every poor country has a version of beans and grains: in Peru, tacu-tacu; in Brazil, feijoada; in Jamaica, dirty rice; in Southern Italy, pasta e fagiole; and so on. By getting protein in this way, you won't be hungry half an hour later.

If you keep your intake of meat down to two ounces a day, it is not necessary to be strictly vegetarian on your "meatless" days. A combination of vegetarian meals and low-meat meals is even better than going vegetarian every other day, because it further reduces intake of cholesterol and animal fat. I have included here some of my favorite recipes that have a bit of meat as a flavoring.

List of Recipes

Brunch

Apple Bran Muffins
Low-Fat Muffins
Egg-Beater Omelet
Potato Frittata (Kugel)

Mostly Vegetarian Main Dishes

Barley Stuffed Peppers
Grilled Portobello Mushroom Steak Burger
Afghan Spinach with Lamb [non-vegetarian]
Spiced Potatoes with Coriander
Banana-Leaf Vegetable Curry
Feijoada (Brazilian Black Beans) [non-vegetarian]
Madras Vegetables

Pasta and Rice

Dad's Vegetarian Pasta with Beans
Pasta with Spinach
Pad Thai Noodles (Easy Version)
Singapore Chow Mein Fun (Curried Noodles)
Korean Noodles with vegetables
Mediterranean-Style Vegetable Lasagne
Baked Tomatoes with Pasta [non-vegetarian]
Herbed Garbanzos and Parsley with Penne
Risotto and Squash Bake
Vegetarian Paella

Side Dishes and Salads

Spicy Okra and Tomato Sauté
Grilled Vegetables
Fried Green Tomatoes with Kaffir Aioli
Rice Pilaf

Thai Cucumber Salad
Winter Fruit Salad

Condiments

Low-Fat Salad Dressing
Thai Sweet and Sour Sauce
Coriander Chutney
Thai Pesto

Soups and Chili

Vegetarian Chili
Mulligatawny Soup
Spicy Thai Shrimp Soup (Tom Yum) [non-vegetarian]

Sweets

Holiday Eggnog
Maple Mousse
Ginger Spice Cookies

Apple Bran Muffins

Ingredients

4 cups flour
3 cups bran
2 teaspoon baking powder
2 teaspoon baking soda
2 teaspoon cinnamon
½ teaspoon nutmeg
1 cup packed brown sugar (to reduce calories,
    substitute Splenda Brown)
¼ cup non-hydrogenated canola margarine
½ cup baby prunes
3 egg whites
14 ounces unsweetened applesauce
1 ½ cup buttermilk or soured milk
½ cup molasses
1 cup raisins
1 apple peeled, chopped
½ cup skim milk powder

Preheat oven to 375°F.
In a medium bowl, whisk together flour, bran, baking powder and soda,
cinnamon, nutmeg, and skim milk powder. In a large bowl cream sugar
and margarine.
Beat in egg whites one at a time until fluffy. Stir in prunes, applesauce,
milk, molasses, raisins, and apple. Add flour mixture and stir until
incorporated.
Spoon batter into paper-lined muffin tin.
Bake for 15–20 min minutes.

Yield: 2 dozen medium-sized muffins

Low-Fat Muffins

Ingredients

1 cup all-purpose flour
2 teaspoons baking powder
1 teaspoon baking soda
½ teaspoon salt
½ teaspoon cinnamon
1 cup oat bran
¼ cup wheat germ
¾ cup sucralose (Splenda)
2 tablespoons crushed flax seed
¼ cup chopped apricots
¾ cup grated carrot
Grated rind of 1 orange
1 cup buttermilk (or milk soured with lemon juice)
2 ounces Egg Beaters
½ cup low-fat yogurt
2 tablespoons canola oil

Preheat oven to 400°F. Sift together flour, baking soda, baking powder, salt, and cinnamon. Stir in bran, wheat germ, and sugar substitute. Stir in flax seeds, apricots, grated carrot, and orange rind. Beat buttermilk, egg substitute, oil, and low-fat yogurt together; pour into dry ingredients and stir to moisten. Fill muffin cups and bake 20 minutes.
Variations: Use applesauce, raisins, cranberries, etc. Nuts are good but high in calories.

Yield: 12 large muffins

Egg Beater Omelet

Ingredients

4 ounces egg substitute (Egg Beaters or Better
    than Eggs), thawed in advance
1 tablespoon each of finely chopped red and green pepper
2 tablespoons chopped green onion
1 tablespoon chopped mushrooms
¼ teaspoon Italian spice
¼ teaspoon black pepper
¼ teaspoon mustard powder
Canola oil or nonstick spray (Pam)

Stir Egg Beaters, mix in spices, and beat until bubbly. Put some canola oil or spray nonstick spray into a nonstick omelet pan. Sauté the veggies with the lid on, then turn heat to low and pour egg mixture into pan. Scrape bottom with spatula repeatedly until egg mixture begins to thicken. Cover until mixture firms up, turning or flipping once while cooking. Serving suggestion: Serve with low-fat sour cream and guacamole on the side. Garnish with sprigs of cilantro.
Variations: Add a bit of cheese while the omelet is thickening; add cilantro and hot peppers (serrano and/or ancho chili powder), or Cajun spice.

Yield: 1 serving

Potato Frittata (Kugel)

Ingredients

Potatoes (as many as you can fit in one layer in a large deep frying pan)
1 large Vidalia onion
2 teaspoons minced garlic
½ cup each green and red bell pepper
1 tablespoon canola oil
Pepper and hot pepper flakes to taste
1 cup soy protein Parmesan cheese
8 ounces thawed egg substitute (such as Egg
    Beaters or Better than Eggs)

Grate the potato (unpeeled) and finely chop the onion and bell peppers. Heat the canola oil and spread around the frying pan. Heat the oven to 350°F. Sauté the onion, garlic, and peppers. Stir in the grated potatoes, then the Egg-Beaters. Add pepper and hot pepper flakes. Stir in half the parmesan cheese and sprinkle the rest on top. Bake for 1 hour, let rest 5 minutes. Serve hot or cold.

Accompaniments: Hot sauce, chutney, or chili sauce
Variations: If diabetes or weight is an issue, use vegetables other than potatoes, such as parsnip, carrots, zucchini, onions, or eggplant. There are hundreds of variants of frittata; this is just one example.

Yield: 6 to 8 servings

Barley Stuffed Peppers

Ingredients

1 cup barley
2 envelopes low-salt vegetable broth
2 tablespoons chopped parsley
1 large onion
1½ cups cheddar cheese
3 medium carrots
2 cans Italian-style tomatoes
2 tablespoons canola oil
2 medium red peppers
1 cup frozen peas
2 medium green peppers
2 medium yellow peppers

In large pan on high heat, bring to boil 3¼ cups water, barley, and broth. Reduce heat, cover, and simmer 1 hour until liquid is absorbed and barley is tender. Meanwhile chop onion and shred carrots. Heat oil in skillet over medium heat and cook onion until tender. Stir in carrots and cook 5 minutes until vegetables are tender and lightly browned. When barley is done, stir in onion mixture, frozen peas, parsley, 1 cup shredded cheese. Set mixture aside.
Preheat oven to 350°F. In a blender, blend tomatoes until almost smooth. Pour into a shallow casserole. Cut top off each pepper and remove seeds. Cut a thin slice from bottom of each pepper so that they will stand straight. Fill peppers with barley mixture and place in casserole. Sprinkle with remaining cheese. Bake 1 hour until tender; cover with foil during the last half hour to prevent overbrowning.

Yield: 6 stuffed peppers

Grilled Portobello Mushroom Steak Burger

Recipe courtesy of food editor Lucy Waverman. I usually allow two mushrooms topped with the cheese and tomato confit per serving, but if they are very large mushrooms, one will be enough. This is more like a steak than a burger.

Ingredients

3 tablespoons olive oil
2 tablespoons balsamic vinegar
2 teaspoons minced garlic
2 shallots, finely chopped
1 tablespoon Dijon mustard
8 portobello mushrooms
Salt and freshly ground pepper

Tomato Confit
2 tablespoons olive oil
¼ cup finely chopped shallots
1 teaspoon minced garlic
2 cups drained chopped canned tomatoes
2 tablespoons fresh basil chopped

½ cup grated Pecorino (Romano) cheese
1 small focaccia bread cut in 8 pieces

Combine oil, vinegar, garlic, shallots, and mustard in a bowl. Brush over mushrooms. Season with salt and pepper to taste. Marinate for one hour. Heat oil in pan on medium high heat. Add shallots and cook for 2 minutes or until softened. Add garlic and tomatoes and cook for 5 minutes, stirring often. Add the basil. Sauce should be thick. Set aside. Preheat barbecue or broiler to high. Grill mushrooms 3 to 4 minutes per side or until browned and tender. Place one mushroom on each piece of focaccia. Top with tomato confit and cheese.

Yield: 4 servings

Afghan Spinach with Lamb
[non-vegetarian]

I figured out a version of this dish after trying it at Pamir, an Afghan restaurant in Guelph, Ontario. Frozen boneless lamb works fine here; just thaw it enough to cut a piece off the end, and refreeze the rest. Frozen ground lamb is also fine in this recipe. Delicious served over basmati rice with coriander chutney.

Ingredients

1 bunch fresh spinach, washed and stemmed (or about
    4 cups of loosely packed baby spinach)
1 medium onion chopped
4 green onions
1 green pepper
6 ounces lamb, cubed
10 cloves cardamom
¼ teaspoon mustard seeds
¼ teaspoon cumin seeds
½ teaspoon hot pepper flakes
Juice of 1 lime

Chop the veggies; grind/blend the spices (I use an old coffee grinder, but a mortar and pestle is the classic way). Brown the lamb and set it aside in a small bowl. Put the veggies in the pan and sauté them. Add the spices, stir, return lamb to pan, and cook until veggies are soft. Add some liquid (e.g., a bit of balsamic vinegar or lime juice) to the pan to deglaze. Place spinach in large casserole; pour lamb mixture on top; squeeze lime juice over the top, cover, and heat in microwave for about 4 minutes, just to soften the spinach but not to overcook.

Yield: 4 to 6 servings, depending on amount of rice and accompaniments

Spiced Potatoes with Coriander

This recipe is modified from a potato salad in Martha Rose Shulman's *Spice of Vegetarian Cooking*. It can be served cold as a salad, but I prefer it hot as a vegetarian main course.

Ingredients

2 pounds red waxy or new potatoes
1 pound ripe tomatoes, diced
4 green onions, minced
1 teaspoon minced garlic
⅓ cup chopped cilantro, including stems
1 teaspoon roasted cumin
Juice of 1–2 lemons or limes, to taste
Salt and pepper to taste
¼ teaspoon hot pepper flakes or cayenne (optional)

Steam the potatoes until tender, about 15 minutes if small; slice into halves or ¼-inch slices depending on size. Put into nonstick pan with a bit of canola oil; stir in the onions, garlic, cilantro and stems; sauté until fragrant. Stir in the tomatoes and sauté until hot, and serve.

Yield: 8 servings

Banana-Leaf Vegetable Curry

Adapted from Sheila Lukins's *All Around the World Cookbook*, this recipe comes from the Banana Leaf Restaurant, Singapore. At the Banana Leaf, instead of a plate and placemat, you get a placemat-sized piece of banana leaf; you discover it's your plate when they come around with buckets of rice and curry and plunk some down on your banana leaf!

Ingredients

1 large onion, chopped
2 tablespoons minced garlic
1½ tablespoons curry powder
6 medium carrots
3 potatoes
1 medium head of cauliflower
4 cups vegetable broth
2 tablespoons honey
1 cinnamon stick
1 19-ounce can chickpeas
½ cup golden raisins
2 cups plum tomatoes
½ cup chopped cilantro
1 cup toasted coconut, for garnish

Peel and dice potatoes; peel carrots, slice in half, then cut into 1-inch pieces; separate cauliflower into florets. Spray nonstick wok and sauté onions until wilted; add garlic, stir for 2–3 minutes. Add curry powder, stir for 2 minutes. Add veggies, broth, honey, and cinnamon stick. Boil, reduce to simmer, and cook uncovered until veggies are tender (20 minutes). Add chickpeas and raisins; simmer 15 minutes, stirring occasionally. Raisins should be just plump. Just before serving, stir in the tomatoes and cilantro and heat through.
Serving suggestions: Serve on basmati rice; garnish with toasted coconut.

Yield: 4 to 7 servings

Feijoada (Brazilian Black Beans) [non-vegetarian]

Ingredients

2 pounds dried black beans
1 tablespoon canola oil
4 cups chopped onion
2 sausages cut into ½-inch slices (try hot Italian
     sausage, chorizo, or other spicy sausage)
4 heaping teaspoons minced garlic
2 teaspoons cumin powder
1 teaspoon mustard powder
6 cups water
½ teaspoon salt
½ teaspoon coarsely ground pepper
1 bay leaf
½ cup red wine vinegar
½ teaspoon hot sauce (or hot pepper flakes)

Sort and wash beans; place in large Dutch oven, cover 2 inches with
water, bring to a boil, and boil 2 minutes. Cover and let stand 1 hour.
Drain and set aside. Wipe pot with paper towel, heat oil in it, and add
onion, sausage, and garlic. Sauté 10 minutes until the onion is tender;
add cumin and mustard; sauté 1 minute. Return beans, add 6 cups water
and spices, and bring to a boil. Cover and simmer for 70 minutes or until
tender. Remove bay leaf, stir in vinegar/hot sauce, and serve on rice.

Yield: 15 cups.

Madras Vegetables

This recipe is modified from Lucy Waverman's *Fast and Fresh Cookbook.*

Ingredients

1 tablespoon minced ginger
½ tablespoon minced garlic
2 tablespoons curry powder
2 potatoes
3 cups cauliflower florets
1 sweet potato
1 cup frozen peas, defrosted
½ cup raisins
⅓ bunch fresh cilantro
½ cup lentils

Dice potatoes and sweet potato, chop cilantro stems, and mince garlic and ginger. Separate cilantro leaves from stems; chop stems; set leaves aside. Spray non-stick pan and sauté garlic, ginger, cilantro stems, and curry powder. Add 1–2 tablespoons water to make paste. Stir in potatoes, lentils, and cauliflower; cover with water (2 inches.), and bring to boil. Cover, reduce heat, and simmer 20 minutes. Add peas and raisins; cook uncovered 5 minutes or until tender. Stir in cilantro leaves and serve. **Serving suggestion:** Serve with rice pilaf.

Yield: 4 to 6 servings

Pasta with Spinach

This is a low-fat variation of a recipe from *La Vera Cucina Italiana*. (The original called for 6 tablespoons of butter! Cornstarch and water can cover a multitude of sins.)

Ingredients

Pasta of choice, about 8 ounces
1 onion
1 green pepper
3 green onions
1 teaspoon minced ginger
1 teaspoon minced garlic
1 cup vegetable (or chicken) broth
⅓ cup hot pepper flakes
1 teaspoon olive oil
Nonstick spray
1 forkful of cornstarch stirred into ½ cup hot water

Chop veggies. Heat large pot of water with a teaspoon of olive oil added. Spray nonstick wok. Sauté veggies, add spices, then add chicken broth. Bring to a boil; add spinach on top to soften in steam. When the spinach is soft, add cornstarch/water to thicken. Add pasta to boiling water in the large pot and cook about 8 minutes, depending on the type of pasta. Reduce the sauce to the right texture and remove from heat. Drain pasta in large colander and toss with the spinach sauce.

Variations: Add more veggies (celery, zucchini), ginger, cumin, cardamom, curry powder, lemon juice, a couple of shrimp per person, etc.

Yield: 2 to 3 servings; for more increase the pasta

Dad's Vegetarian Pasta with Beans

Ingredients

1 lb (450 gram) package whole-grain pasta of choice
½–1 green pepper
4 green onions
½ large onion
1 tablespoon minced ginger
1 shallot
2 teaspoons minced garlic
½ cup celery
¾ cup chickpeas and/or black beans (canned, frozen, or precooked)
1 teaspoon Italian spice
1 tablespoon cornstarch
½ teaspoon hot pepper flakes

Put a large pot of water on to boil and add about a teaspoon of olive oil. Chop pepper and onions. Finely mince the garlic, ginger, and shallot. (You can save time by using prechopped ginger and garlic, or paste.) Spray a nonstick wok and sauté veggies and spices. Put the cornstarch in a cup, stirring vigorously while running enough hot water into cup from tap to make a thin paste; add cornstarch/water to wok to thicken sauce. Turn off heat and stir occasionally to prevent excessive thickening; add a bit of water as needed to adjust thickness.
Add pasta to pot when water reaches a rolling boil; stir several times early on to prevent sticking. At about 8 minutes, depending on the shape of the pasta (or about 3 minutes for fresh pasta), drain in a large colander, then toss in the wok with the tasty veggie sauce.

Serving suggestions: Serve with a bit of grated cheese, and a crusty roll or garlic bread.
Variations: Add chopped cilantro or a bit of coriander chutney; use tomato sauce, mushrooms, different kinds of beans, chopped carrots, or Hoisin sauce.

Yield: 4 to 6 servings

Pad Thai Noodles (Easy Version)

Ingredients

1½ pound package flat rice noodles
1 cup green beans
1 cup carrots
1 cup green onions
4 ounces Szechuan peanut sauce (such as President's
    Choice Memories of Szechuan brand)
4 ounces spicy tamarind sauce (such as President's
    Choice Memories of Bangkok brand)
½ teaspoon hot pepper flakes
½ cup fresh cilantro

Put water on to boil in large pot. Julienne beans, carrots, and onions. Spray nonstick wok ; sauté veggies. Add pepper flakes. Stir sauces into veggies. Put noodles into boiling water, remove from stove, and after 5 minutes drain into large colander. Toss with veggies and sauce.

Serving suggestion: Serve in bowls; sprinkle with fresh cilantro and crushed peanuts.
Variations: Add about 8–10 leaves of chopped fresh basil; put some large chunks of lemon grass in the pasta water before boiling and fish them out of the colander before serving; add a few chopped shrimps to fancy up this dish.
Substitutions: If you can't find President's Choice or similar sauces, as a substitute for the peanut sauce, stir a forkful of cornstarch into a cup of hot water and then stir in a tablespoon of peanut butter. As a substitute for the tamarind sauce, try Sheila Lukins's Thai Sweet and Sour Sauce in the condiment section.

Yield: 6 servings

Singapore Chow Mein Fun (Curried Noodles)

Ingredients

3 green onions
½ green pepper
½ red bell pepper
½ medium onion
½ cup peas
1 teaspoon minced garlic
½ teaspoon minced ginger
⅓ cup fresh cilantro
Juice of 1 lime
2 tablespoons curry powder
1 teaspoon mustard powder
½ teaspoon hot pepper flakes
1 forkful cornstarch
1 cup hot water
8 ounces whole grain pasta (linguine works well, but any pasta is fine)

Chop the onions and peppers. Stir the cornstarch into the water. Put a large pot of water on to boil for pasta, with a teaspoon of olive oil in it. Spray nonstick wok and put it on medium heat. Sauté peppers and onions until the onions are limp. Add the garlic and ginger; stir and cook another minute. Add the curry powder; stir and cook another minute. Add the hot pepper flakes and mustard powder, cook briefly; then stir in the cornstarch and water, and the lime juice. Bring to a boil and remove from heat, stirring occasionally.
Cook the pasta according to package directions; drain; adjust the thickness of the sauce (add a little water or white wine if it's too thick; cook a bit longer if it's not thick enough). Put the pasta into the wok and toss with sauce. Serve.

Variations: Add 2 ounces chopped ham or back bacon and a couple of medium shrimp chopped into quarter-inch pieces.

Yield: 4 servings; for more increase the pasta

Korean Noodles with Vegetables

A good vegetarian main course from Lucy Waverman.

Ingredients

6 ounces Korean glass noodles or rice sticks
2 tablespoons light soy sauce
2 teaspoons sugar or sucralose (Splenda)
2 teaspoons sesame oil
2 tablespoons vegetable oil
1 tablespoon minced garlic
2 teaspoons minced ginger
6 shiitake mushrooms, thinly sliced
1 cup julienne carrot
1 cup thinly sliced onion
4 cups baby spinach
1 cup Chinese chives, cut in 3-inch lengths
Salt and freshly ground pepper to taste
2 tablespoons green onion, chopped
2 tablespoons sesame seeds

Boil a large pot of water. Add noodles and boil for 4 minutes or until transparent and softened but still with a little texture. Drain and rinse with cold water. Set aside.
Combine soy sauce, sugar and sesame oil in a mixing bowl.
Heat wok on high heat and add vegetable oil. Add garlic and ginger and stir fry for 30 seconds. Toss in mushrooms, carrot, and onion and stir fry for 1 minute, or until slightly softened. Add spinach and cook until just wilted. Stir in chives and noodles and mix together. Stir in soy sauce mixture and season well. Serve with green onions and sesame seeds.

Yield: 2 servings

Mediterranean-Style Vegetable Lasagne

A quick and flavorful lasagne using seasonal vegetables from food editor Lucy Waverman. Look for Sicilian eggplant if available, it has a soft, custard-like texture and no bitterness. The instant, dried lasagne noodles are available in boxes at the supermarket. Although they can be used without any pre-soaking, they soften more easily if you soak them for a couple of minutes in water before using.

Ingredients

2 tablespoons olive oil
1 large onion, diced
1 teaspoon minced garlic
2 small zucchini, diced
½ eggplant, peeled and diced
1 red pepper, diced
1 teaspoon dried basil
½ teaspoon red pepper flakes or more to taste
1 can tomatoes (28 ounces/796 ml.), pureed
¼ cup black olives, pitted and sliced
¼ cup chopped parsley
Salt and freshly ground pepper
8 ounces fontina, provolone, mozzarella, or cheddar, grated
1 cup Parmesan cheese, grated
9 instant lasagne noodles

Heat olive oil in large skillet over medium heat. Add onion and garlic and sauté until onion is softened slightly. Add zucchini, eggplant and pepper and cook 5 minutes longer. Sprinkle with basil and pepper flakes. Add tomatoes, stir together and simmer, covered, for 15 minutes. Stir in olives and parsley and season with salt and pepper. Set aside.
Combine fontina and Parmesan cheese.
Preheat oven to 375°F. In a buttered 7 x 11-inch gratin dish, layer one third lasagne noodles, slightly overlapping, one third of sauce, and one third of cheese. Repeat two more layers finishing with sauce and cheese. Bake 30 minutes or until sauce is bubbling and cheese is melted. Let set for about 15 minutes before serving.

Yield: 4 to 6 servings

Baked Tomatoes with Pasta [non-vegetarian]

This rustic dish from Lucy Waverman is perfect for flavorful summer tomatoes. Use less anchovy, if desired.

Ingredients

6 beefsteak tomatoes
¼ cup olive oil
1 can anchovy fillets
1 tablespoon minced garlic
1 teaspoon chopped fresh thyme
2 tablespoons slivered basil
Salt and freshly ground pepper
1 pound whole wheat penne pasta
Freshly grated Parmesan cheese

Preheat oven to 400°F.
Slice tomatoes thickly. Oil an ovenproof baking sheet with 1 tablespoons oil. Place one layer tomatoes on sheet. Top with half of anchovy filets, half of garlic and herbs. Season layer with salt and pepper. Add a second layer on top with remaining anchovy, garlic and herbs. Pour over remaining 3 tablespoons olive oil. Bake for 30 minutes.
Remove from oven and coarsely chop up tomatoes using kitchen scissors. Return to baking dish and bake for 30 minutes longer or until juices have thickened slightly and sauce has lots of taste.
Boil pasta according to package directions. Drain and toss with tomatoes. Serve with Parmesan.

Yield: 6 to 8 servings

Herbed Garbanzos and Parsley with Penne

This recipe is modified from a recipe on Bob's Red Mill website.

Ingredients

2 cups cooked/canned garbanzo beans (chickpeas)
2 teaspoons olive oil
1 medium red onion
2 cloves garlic, minced (or 1½ teaspoons garlic paste)
Zest of 1 lemon
1 teaspoon ground cumin
¼ teaspoon oregano
¼ teaspoon salt
¼ teaspoon chili pepper, chipotle (ground)
1 pound penne pasta
1 cup fresh chopped parsley
3 tablespoons fresh lemon juice
1 cup vegetable stock

In a large nonstick skillet, heat oil over medium heat; add the onion and garlic, cover and cook until the onions are browned, about 5 minutes. Add the cooked garbanzo beans, stock, lemon zest and juice, cumin, oregano, salt and hot chili pepper. Cover, reduce the heat to low, and simmer for 5 minutes. Meanwhile, in a large pot of boiling, salted water, cook the pasta until barely tender, about 7 minutes; do not overcook. Drain and return to the pot. Add the garbanzo mixture and the parsley to the pasta and cook over medium-low heat, stirring gently until the pasta has absorbed most of the liquid, 2–3 minutes. Transfer to a warmed serving bowl and serve immediately.

Yield: 6 to 8 servings

Risotto and Squash Bake

A wonderful vegetarian main dish or side dish using sweet winter squash, adapted from a recipe on Bob's Red Mill website.

Ingredients

1 cup arborio or carnaroli rice (I think carnaroli is better for risotto)
2 tablespoons olive oil
½ cup chopped yellow onion
½ cup chopped mushrooms
3¾ cups vegetable (or chicken) stock, to be divided in thirds
2 cups winter squash, cooked and pureed
1½ cups Parmesan cheese, freshly grated
3 tablespoons low-fat sour cream

Preheat oven to 400°F. In a large, deep ovenproof skillet heat the olive oil and sauté the onion and mushrooms until the onion is soft and yellow. Add the rice and stir to coat with oil. Add 1¼ cups of stock to risotto and place skillet in oven. After 15 minutes add another 1¼ cups of stock to risotto; stir to combine; and place skillet back in oven. In another 15 minutes add the last 1¼ cups of stock and the squash to risotto. Bake for 15 minutes; add the low-fat sour cream and cheese; return the skillet to the oven to bake for an additional 15 minutes. Serve immediately.

Yield: 6 to 8 servings as a main course

Vegetarian Paella

Ingredients

1 tablespoon oil
1 large onion, chopped
2 teaspoon minced garlic
1 cup long grain rice
½ teaspoon ground turmeric
½ teaspoon ground cumin
¼ teaspoon ground cinnamon
1 cup frozen corn
1 14-ounce can unsalted tomatoes
1 cup frozen peas
1 can kidney beans, drained
½ cup seedless raisins
¼ cup sliced almonds, toasted
Generous pinch of saffron (if you can afford it)

Sauté onion in oil for 3 minutes. Add garlic and sauté 1 minute. Stir in rice, turmeric (and saffron), cumin, and cinnamon. Drain tomatoes and set tomatoes aside. Add enough water to drained tomato juice to make 1¾ cup. Add to skillet and bring to a boil. Lower heat, cover, and simmer for 10 minutes. Stir in thawed corn, peas, beans, drained tomatoes, and raisins. Cover and simmer 10 minutes or until the rice is tender and the liquid is absorbed. Serve with almonds sprinkled on top.

Yield: 6 servings

Spicy Okra and Tomato Sauté

This recipe is modified slightly from Martha Rose Shulman's *Spice of Vegetarian Cooking*.

Ingredients

1 tablespoon canola oil
1 large onion, chopped
2 teaspoons minced garlic
2 teaspoons sweet paprika
1 hot green chili pepper, chopped
1 pound okra, trimmed and sliced
½ inch thick (discard the ends)
1 tablespoon wine vinegar
3 tablespoons white wine
1 pound tomatoes, fresh or canned, sliced
1 tablespoon chopped cilantro or basil
Salt and pepper to taste

Heat the oil in a large heavy pan or casserole; add the onion and half the garlic and sauté on medium heat until onion begins to soften. Add paprika and chili pepper; sauté a few minutes more, stirring. Add okra and vinegar; sauté until bright green (about 5 minutes). Add wine, tomatoes, and remaining garlic; cook 10–15 minutes, stirring occasionally, until okra is tender and mixture aromatic. Add basil or coriander; season to taste.

Serving suggestions: Serve with hot cooked grains such as bulgur, brown rice, barley, lentils, or a mixture. Barley and brown rice, about half and half, make a nice combination: bring 2 cups of water to a boil, add 1 cup of grains, and cook on low for 30 minutes.

Yield: 6 servings

Grilled Vegetables

Ingredients *(vary quantities as desired)*

Chop into large chunks
large onion (or pearl onions)
green and red pepper
yellow zucchini
portabella mushroom
baby carrots
Toss in
    baby carrots
    eggplant slices

Marinate vegetables in ¼ cup light soya sauce with ¼ cup balsamic vinegar, 1 teaspoon mustard powder, ½ teaspoon hot pepper flakes, 1 teaspoon sesame oil, freshly ground pepper. Grill on barbecue using a grilling basket; serve with boiled new potatoes (or throw parboiled new potatoes into the basket).

Fried Green Tomatoes with Kaffir Aioli

This recipe was given to me by Ryan Hermann, chef at The Fish Restaurant in Charleston, South Carolina. Although this is not a low-fat recipe, if you use canola oil for the frying, you will be adding beneficial fat to your diet.

Ingredients

The sauce:
Egg substitute (equivalent to 1 egg)
Cayenne pepper (optional)
¼ teaspoon salt
3 teaspoons fresh lemon juice
6 kaffir lime leaves, chopped
1 cup good olive

2 firm bright green tomatoes
flour for dredging
canola oil for frying

The tempura batter:
2 cups flour
Salt and pepper, a couple of shakes
1 ½ cups club soda

Combine all sauce ingredients except oil in a blender, and puree. Add the oil slowly—it should thicken as you go. Taste it and adjust for seasoning; add a little cayenne pepper if you like it spicy. Set the aioli aside.
Slice the tomatoes a quarter inch thick. Dredge them lightly in flour, and then in the tempura batter. Fry them in canola oil. At 350°F, one minute on each side. When done they will be crispy and golden brown. Pat them dry and salt them lightly, and serve with the kaffir aioli.

Note: Kaffir lime leaves are readily available at Asian markets and finer grocery stores. If you can't find them, substitute finely chopped zest a lime. Alternatively, substitute cilantro and lime juice for the kaffir and lemon juice.

Yield: 4 servings

Rice Pilaf

This recipe is modified from Lucy Waverman's *Fast and Fresh Cookbook.*

Ingredients

2 cups basmati rice
2 cups water
1 teaspoon turmeric (pinch of saffron)
6 cloves
1 teaspoon cumin seeds
2 bay leaves
½ cinnamon stick
Salt to taste

Soak rice 30 minutes, drain, and put in heavy pot with 2 cups water and remaining ingredients. Bring to a boil, stir in 1 tablespoon olive oil, cover, and reduce heat to low. Cook 15 minutes. Remove from heat, uncover, and stir.

Variation: Stir in finely chopped onions fried to brown and some finely grated carrot.

Yield: 6 to 8 servings

Thai Cucumber Salad

Ingredients

⅓ cup shallots
⅓ cup green onions
4 medium cucumbers
2–4 small hot red chili peppers
½ cup rice vinegar
2 tablespoons sugar or sucralose (Splenda)
¼ teaspoon salt
¼ cup chopped cilantro

Mince shallots and slice green onions. Pee cucumbers, cut them in half lengthwise, seed, and slice into thin slices. Slice the hot peppers open lengthwise, remove the seeds, and slice very thinly. Combine cucumbers, onions, shallots, and peppers in a large bowl. Combine sugar, vinegar, and salt; add to cucumber mix and toss well. Stir in the cilantro and serve.

Yield: 10 half-cup servings

Side Dishes and Salads

Winter Fruit Salad

Winter fruits make an excellent salad when they are marinated with a tasty dressing. Blood oranges are available from late January through April and their intense ruby color makes an attractive dressing. This recipe is courtesy of Lucy Waverman.

Ingredients

2 blood or navel oranges
2 bananas
1 cantaloupe
3 kiwi fruit
1 cup seedless red or green grapes

Dressing:
½ cup blood orange juice
1 tablespoon sugar
1 tablespoon chopped preserved ginger or to taste
1 tablespoon lime juice
1 teaspoon ground cardamom

Peel oranges removing all the white pith and cut into sections. Peel and thinly slice bananas. Scoop cantaloupe into balls with melon baller. Alternatively, the melon can be diced. Peel and thinly slice kiwi fruit. Toss with grapes. Arrange attractively in large glass bowl.
For the dressing combine blood orange juice, sugar, ginger, lime juic,e and cardamom in small bowl. Drizzle over salad and chill thoroughly before serving.

Yield: 6 servings

Low-Fat Salad Dressing

This has about one-third the calories and fat of a regular vinaigrette.

Ingredients

¼ cup vinegar (or juice of 1 lime)
¼ cup olive oil
½ cup water less 1 tablespoon
1 teaspoon cornstarch
1 teaspoon mustard powder
½ teaspoon Italian spice
½ teaspoon coarsely ground pepper

Add mustard powder and spices to vinegar. Stir cornstarch into water. Cook in microwave for a minute or two to thicken. After the spices have steeped in the vinegar for a few minutes, add the olive oil and thickened cornstarch/water, and beat briskly.
Variations: Balsamic vinegar, fresh basil leaves, fresh coriander, fresh oregano, ½ teaspoon of mustard seeds.

Yield: 1 cup

Thai Sweet and Sour Sauce

From Sheila Lukins's *All Around the World Cookbook*. For making the Pad Thai noodles recipe, run this through a food processor or blender. It will keep for a while in the fridge.

Ingredients

1 cup rice wine vinegar
½ cup water
½ cup sugar or sucralose (Splenda)
½ cup light brown sugar
1–2 teaspoons chopped fresh red chilies
1 teaspoon salt
1 teaspoon minced garlic 1 teaspoon chopped cilantro
    stems and roots, strings removed (wash carefully)
1 cup seeded, and chopped cucumber
1 tablespoon cilantro leaves, for garnish

Combine vinegar, water, sugars, chilis, salt, garlic, and chopped cilantro stems in a saucepan; cook over low heat 2 minutes, stirring. Remove to bowl and let cool. Stir in the cucumber and cilantro leaves; serve or refrigerate immediately.

Yield: 2 cups

Coriander Chutney

I discovered this wonderful mixture in Pamir, an Afghan restaurant in Guelph, Ontario, and then found that it is sold at the Indian grocery store around the corner. A great addition to chili on rice and other dishes.

Ingredients

1 large bunch of fresh cilantro
Juice of 1 large or 2 small limes
¼ teaspoon hot pepper flakes
¼ teaspoon salt (or a teaspoon of soy sauce)

Wash cilantro carefully. Remove strings from roots, then chop coarsely including roots and stems, and place in a food processor or blender. Add lime juice and hot peppers, blend, and serve. If it's too thick, add a bit more lime juice or a bit of balsamic vinegar.
Variations: Add a bit of fresh mint.

Yield: about 1 cup

Thai Pesto

My daughter-in-law, Kate Gutteridge, a fine gardener, made up this recipe to use up some of her cilantro before it went to seed. It's a very easy way to make a quick delicious pasta dish, can be prepared up to a few days ahead, and will keep in the fridge for a while. Just toss with cooked pasta and serve. (It's also okay to use cilantro after it has gone to seed; throw the flowers in too!)

Ingredients

3 heaping teaspoons minced garlic
2 tablespoons minced ginger
1 bunch fresh cilantro, roots removed
¼ cup dry-roasted peanuts
½ teaspoon crushed red pepper
½ cup canola oil
4 green onions, chopped

With food processor running, drop garlic and ginger through tube. Add cilantro, peanuts, and red pepper. Gradually add oil. Season to taste with salt.

Yield: about a cup

Vegetarian Chili

Ingredients

1 can tomatoes (14 ounces)
1 can tomato juice (about 14 ounces)
1 large can kidney beans (about 28 ounces/800 ml)
1 can low-fat refried beans (about 7 ounces)
1 green pepper
4 green onions
1 medium onion
1 cup chopped celery with tops
1 cup chopped carrots
1 tablespoon cumin powder
4 tablespoons chili powder
1 tablespoon mustard powder
¼–½ teaspoon hot chili flakes
Coarsely ground pepper
2 tablespoons balsamic vinegar
A bit of salt if you must (or light soy sauce)
Canola oil

Chop onions, celery, carrots, and green pepper; sauté with a minimum of spray or canola oil in a large nonstick pot or electric frying pan. Add spices and stir. Add tomatoes and kidney beans, stir, and simmer while the rice is cooking. Thicken with low-fat refried beans.

Serving suggestions: Serve on brown rice or barley and rice. Add hot sauce to taste, a little coriander chutney (see recipe), and a few drops of sesame oil to raise this dish to gourmet status. Freeze the leftovers in portion-sized freezer bags to reheat in the microwave.
Variations: Add or substitute chickpeas, frozen corn kernels, red pepper, etc.

Yield: 8 to 10 servings

Mulligatawny Soup

This recipe is adapted from Martha Rose Shulman's *Spice of Vegetarian Cooking*.

Ingredients

2 tablespoons canola oil
2 tablespoons curry powder
1 onion, minced
2 teaspoons minced ginger
2 carrots, minced
½ cup raw or unsalted peanuts
2 green peppers, chopped
2 quarts vegetable stock
4 whole cloves
½ cup almonds, coarsely chopped in a blender
1 tablespoon honey
2 tablespoons shredded coconut
½ cup raisins
2 tart apples, peeled and diced
4 whole cloves
1 teaspoon ground mace or nutmeg
3 tomatoes, peeled and chopped
1½ cups cooked brown rice
1 apple, sliced thin, for garnish

Heat the oil in a large heavy soup pot; sauté the onion with curry powder, ginger, apples, carrots, peanuts, and green pepper for about 3 minutes or until onion starts to soften. Add the vegetable stock, cloves, almonds, honey, coconut, raisins, mace/nutmeg, salt, pepper, and tomatoes; bring to simmer. Cover and simmer on low for 30 minutes. Remove half the soup and puree in a blender; return to pot and stir well. Heat through, adjust seasonings, and stir in the cooked brown rice.

Serving suggestion: Top each bowl with a couple of thin slices of apple. Can be served cold as a salad, but I prefer it hot as a vegetarian main course.

Yield: 6 to 8 servings

Spicy Thai Shrimp Soup (Tom Yum) [non-vegetarian]

One of the nicest Christmas presents I ever got was a complete kit to make Tom Yum soup. My son Jeff and daughter-in-law Kate Gutteridge put it together for me, knowing how I love it. They included a recipe, and it's now one of our regulars.

Ingredients

⅓ cup shallots
¼ cup roughly chopped lemon grass
1 tablespoon minced ginger
1 teaspoon minced garlic
1 tablespoon chopped Cilantro stems
Nonstick spray
3 medium shrimp, halved lengthwise, per person (up to about 12)
6 cups water
1 can straw or button mushrooms
3 tablespoons fresh lime juice
1 tablespoon Thai fish sauce
¼ teaspoon chili oil
¼ cup chopped fresh cilantro

Heat nonstick pan and add first five ingredients. Sauté 2 minutes, set aside. Spray pan, heat, add shrimp; sauté 3 minutes, set aside. Boil water in pot, add shallot/ginger/cilantro/lemon-grass mix, simmer 10 minutes.

Serving suggestion: Lift out the lemon-grass chunks; spoon mixture into bowls, ensuring that each has some shrimp and mushrooms; sprinkle chopped cilantro on top.
Variations: The lemon grass is important, but if you can't find it this is still a good soup. Use minced galangal, the Thai ginger, if you can find it. There is a paste available in Thai grocery stores called Canh Chua Thailan (sour soup paste) that is used to make this soup in Thai homes and restaurants; it isn't perfect as it contains palm oil, but there's not a lot of oil in it and it is authentic; I use a couple of teaspoons in a batch.

Yield: 4 to 6 servings

Holiday Eggnog

Not as cloyingly thick as most commercial eggnogs, this is more like the milk punch served at Brennan's in New Orleans.

Ingredients

1 cup egg substitute
2 cups 1% milk
Sucralose (Splenda) to taste (start with a couple of tablespoons)
1 teaspoon vanilla extract
Sprinkle of ground nutmeg and cinnamon

Combine first four ingredients in a punch bown. Sprinkle with nutmeg and cinnamon.
Variations: add ⅓ cup amber rum, ⅓ cup brandy, and ⅓ cup whisky
For a fancy version, whip 2 egg whites (½ cup) and fold in.

Yield: 6 to 8 servings

Maple Mousse

Adapted from Lucy Waverman's low fat version of a favorite dessert.

Ingredients

2 cups drained low-fat yogurt
½ cup maple syrup
2 tablespoons brandy
1 teaspoon grated lemon rind
2 egg whites
2 teaspoons sucralose (Splenda).

Place yogurt in large bowl. Place maple syrup in a pot over medium heat and reduce until ¼ cup remains. Add brandy. Beat hot mixture into yogurt along with lemon rind.
Beat egg whites until frothy, then beat in sugar. Continue until egg whites hold soft peaks. Fold into yogurt mixture. Spoon into glass dishes and serve with Ginger Spice Cookies.

Yield: 4 servings

Ginger Spice Cookies

A low fat cookie from Lucy Waverman to serve with a creamy dessert.

Ingredients

1 cup all purpose flour
1 teaspoon minced ginger
¼ teaspoon nutmeg
¼ teaspoon cinnamon
¼ teaspoon cloves
¼ cup canola margarine
¼ cup packed brown sugar
¼ cup sucralose (Splenda)
2 ounces egg substitute

Preheat oven to 350°F. Sift together flour, ginger, nutmeg, cinnamon, and cloves.
In a separate bowl, cream margarine and sugar with an electric mixer until light. Beat in egg substitute. Stir in flour mixture until blended.
Gather dough into ball and refrigerate for 1 hour.
Lay half of dough between sheets of plastic wrap and roll out thinly. Cut with cookie cutter into 2-inch rounds. Prick each cookie with a fork. Repeat with remaining dough.
Bake on ungreased cookie sheets for 5 to 7 minutes or until golden. Cool on racks.

Yield: 20 cookies

Some of My Favorite Cookbooks

Casselman, Barbie. *Good-for-You Cookbook: A Healthy Eating Guide.* Toronto: Random House of Canada, 1993.

Lukins, Sheila. *All Around the World Cookbook.* New York: Workman, 1994.

Madison, Deborah (with Edward Espe Brown). *The Greens Cook Book.* New York: Bantam Books, 1987.

Podleski, Janet, and Greta Podleski. *Crazy Plates: Low-Fat Food So Good, You'll Swear It's Bad for You!* New York: Perigee, 2000.

Podleski, Janet, and Greta Podleski.. *Looneyspoons: Low-Fat Food Made Fun.* New York: Perigee, 2000. (Note: Substitute Egg Beaters or egg whites for eggs, canola margarine for butter, and so on, when using the Podleski sisters' books.)

Shulman, Martha Rose. *The Spice of Vegetarian Cooking.* Rochester, Vermont: Healing Arts Press, 1991.

Soviero, Donaldo. *La Vera Cucina Italiana: The Fundamentals of Classic Italian Cooking.* New York: Macmillan, 1991.

Waverman, Lucy. *Home for Dinner.* Toronto: Random House of Canada, 2002.

Waverman, Lucy. *Lucy Waverman's Fast and Fresh Cookbook.* Richmond Hill, Ontario: Firefly Books, 1997.

Internet Sources

www.bobsredmill.com (a source for whole grain recipes)

www.epicurious.com (a source for recipes of all kinds)

www. glycemicindex.com (reference to how quickly foods are converted to sugar)

http://harpercollins.ca/mot (sample recipes from *A Matter of Taste,* by Lucy Waverman and James Chatto)

www.lucywaverman.com (website of Lucy Waverman, Food Editor, *Food & Drink;* Food Columnist, *The Globe & Mail*)

www.nutritiondata.com (calorie counts)

www.ontariobeans.on.ca (recipes and cooking information for beans)

www. recipezaar.com (over 150,000 recipes submitted by subscribers worldwide)

References

(1) Barnett HJM, Taylor DW, Eliasziw M, Fox AJ, Ferguson GG, Haynes RB, et al. Benefit of carotid endarterectomy in patients with symptomatic moderate or severe carotid stenosis. N Engl J Med 1998;339:1415–25.

(2) International Study of Unruptured Intracranial Aneurysms Investigators. Unruptured intracranial aneurysms—risk of rupture and risks of surgical intervention. N Engl J Med 1998;339:1725–33.

(3) Gunel M, Awad IA, Finberg K, Anson JA, Steinberg GK, Batjer HH, et al. A founder mutation as a cause of cerebral cavernous malformation in Hispanic Americans. N Engl J Med 1996;334:946–51.

(4) Beaudry M, Spence JD. Motor vehicle accidents: the most common cause of traumatic vertebrobasilar ischemia. Can J Neurol Sci 2003;30:320–25.

(5) Weintraub MI. Beauty parlor stroke syndrome: report of five cases. JAMA 1993;269:2085–86.

(6) Cherkin DC, Deyo RA, Battie M, Street J, Barlow W. A comparison of physical therapy, chiropractic manipulation, and provision of an educational booklet for the treatment of patients with low back pain. N Engl J Med 1998 Oct 8;339 (15):1021–29.

(7) Hurwitz EL, Morgenstern H, Harber P, Kominski GF, Belin TR, Yu F, et al. A randomized trial of medical care with and without physical therapy and chiropractic care with and without physical modalities for patients with low back pain: 6-month follow-up outcomes from the UCLA low back pain study. Spine 2002 Oct 15;27 (20):2193–204.

(8) Wong DG, Spence JD, Lamki L, McDonald JWD. Effect of non-

steroidal anti-inflammatory drugs on control of hypertension by beta-blockers and diuretics. Lancet i, 997–1001. 1986.

(9)   Spence JD, Hegele RA. Non-invasive assessment of atherosclerosis risk. Curr Drug Targets Cardiovasc Haematol Disord 2004 Jun;4 (2):125–28.

(10)   Spence J.D., Hegele RA. Noninvasive phenotypes of atherosclerosis. Arterioscler Thromb Vasc Biol 2004;24 (11):e188.

(11)   Spence JD, Eliasziw M, DiCicco M, Hackam DG, Galil R, Lohmann T. Carotid plaque area: a tool for targeting and evaluating vascular preventive therapy. Stroke 2002 Dec;33 (12):2916–22.

(12)   Robertson J, Iemolo F, Stabler SP, Allen RH, Spence JD. Vitamin B12, homocysteine and carotid plaque in the era of folic acid fortification of enriched cereal grain products. CMAJ 2005 Jun 7;172 (12):1569–73.

(13)   Ainsworth CD, Blake CC, Tamayo A, Beletsky V, Fenster A, Spence JD. 3D ultrasound measurement of change in carotid plaque volume: a tool for rapid evaluation of new therapies. Stroke 2005 Sep;36 (9):1904–9.

(14)   Fenster A, Landry A, Downey DB, Hegele RA, Spence JD. 3D ultrasound imaging of the carotid arteries. Curr Drug Targets Cardiovasc Haematol Disord 2004 Jun;4 (2):161–75.

(15)   Spence JD. Point: uses of carotid plaque measurement as a predictor of cardiovascular events. Prev Cardiol 2005;8 (2):118–21.

(16)   Executive Committee for the Asymptomatic Carotid Atherosclerosis Study. Endarterectomy for asymptomatic carotid artery stenosis. JAMA 1995;272:1421–28.

(17)   Spence JD, Tamayo A, Lownie SP, Ng W, Ferguson GG. Absence of microemboli on transcranial Doppler identifies low-risk patients with asymptomatic carotid stenosis who do not warrant endarterectomy or stenting. Stroke 2005;36:2373–78.

(18)   Barnett PA, Spence JD, Manuck SB, Jennings JR. Psychological stress and the progression of carotid atherosclerosis. J Hypertension 1997;15:49–55.

(19)   Chimowitz MI, Weiss DG, Cohen SL, Starling MR, Hobson RW 2nd. Cardiac prognosis of patients with carotid stenosis and no history of coronary artery disease. Veterans Affairs Cooperative Study Group 167. Stroke 1994 Apr;25(4):759–65.

(20)   Spence JD. Fasting lipids: the carrot in the snowman. Can J Cardiol 2003;19:890–92.

(21)   Levy Y, Maor I, Presser D, Aviram M. Consumption of eggs with meals increases the susceptibility of human plasma and low-

density lipoprotein to lipid peroxidation. Ann Nutr Metab 1996;40 (5):243–51.

(22) Hu FB, Stampfer MJ, Rimm EB, Manson JE, Ascherio A, Colditz GA, et al. A prospective study of egg consumption and risk of cardiovascular disease in men and women. JAMA 1999 Apr 21;281 (15):1387–94.

(23) De Lorgeril M, Salen P, Martin JL, Monjaud I, Delaye J, Mamelle N. Mediterranean diet, traditional risk factors, and the rate of cardiovascular complications after myocardial infarction: final report of the Lyon Diet Heart Study [see comments]. Circulation 1999 Feb 16;99 (6):779–85.

(24) Singh RB, Dubnov G, Niaz MA, Gosh S, Singh R, Rastogi SS, et al. Effect of an Indo-Mediterranean diet on progression of coronary artery disease in high-risk patients (Indo-Mediterranean Diet Heart Study): a randomized single-blind trial. Lancet 2002;360:1455–61.

(25) Spence JD, Huff MW, Heidenheim P, Viswanatha A, Munoz C, Lindsay R, et al. Combination therapy with colestipol and psyllium mucilloid in patients with hyperlipidemia. Ann Intern Med 1995 Oct 1;123 (7):493–99.

(26) Stern RH, Freeman DJ, Spence JD. Differences in metabolism of time-release and unmodified nicotinic acid: Explanation of the differences in hypolipidemic action? Metabolism 1992;41:879–81.

(27) Brater DC, Morrelli HF. Digoxin toxicity in patients with normokalemic potassium depletion. Clin Pharmacol Ther 1977 Jul 22:21–33.

(28) Spence JD. The current epidemic of primary aldosteronism: causes and consequences. J Hypertens 2004;22:2038–9.

(29) Spence JD. Physiologic tailoring of therapy for resistant hypertension: 20 years' experience with stimulated renin profiling. Am J Hypertens 1999;12:1077–83.

(30) Wallach L, Nyarai I, Dawson KG. Stimulated renin: a screening test for hypertension. Ann Int Med 1975;82:27–34.

(31) Laragh JH. Modern system for treating high blood pressure based on renin profiling and vasoconstriction-volume analysis: a primary role for beta blocking drugs such as propranolol. Am J Med 1976;61:797–810.

(32) Baker EH, Duggal A, Dong Y, Ireson NJ, Wood M, Markandu ND, et al. Amiloride, a specific drug for hypertension in black people with T594M variant? Hypertension 2002;40:13–17.

(33) Grim CE, Robinson M. Salt, slavery and survival—Hypertension in the African diaspora/.Epidemiology 2003 Jan;14(1):120–2.

(34) Rangno RE, Langlois S. Comparison of withdrawal phenomena after propranolol, metoprolol, and pindolol. Am Heart J. 1982 Aug;104(2 Pt 2):473–8.

(35) MacDowall P, Kalra PA, O'Donoghue DJ, Waldek S, Mamtora H, Brown K. Risk of morbidity from renovascular disease in elderly patients with congestive cardiac failure. Lancet 1998 Jul 4;352(9121):13–6.

(36) Brater DC, Morrelli HF. Digoxin toxicity in patients with normokalemic potassium depletion. Clin Pharmacol Ther 1977 Jul 22:21–33.

(37) Spence JD, Wong DG, Lindsay RM. Effects of triamterene and amiloride on urinary sediment in hypertensive patients taking hydrochlorothiazide. Lancet 1985 Jul 13;2 (8446):73–75.

(38) Vladutiu GD, Simmons Z, Isackson PJ, Tarnopolsky M, Peltier WL, Barboi AC, Sripathi N, Wortmann RL, Phillips PS. Genetic risk factors associated with lipid-lowering drug-induced myopathies. Muscle Nerve 2006 May 2.

(39) Results from Kelly et al. are not yet available in print.

(40) Andres E, Loukili NH, Noel E, Kaltenbach G, Abdelgheni MB, Perrin AE, et al. Vitamin B12 (cobalamin) deficiency in elderly patients. CMAJ 2004 Aug 3;171 (3):251–59.

(41) Schnyder G, Roffi M, Pin R, Flammer Y, Lange H, Eberli FR, et al. Decreased rate of coronary restenosis after lowering of plasma homocysteine levels. N Engl J Med 2001;345 (22):1593–600.

(42) Schnyder G, Roffi M, Flammer Y, Pin R, Hess OM. Effect of homocysteine-lowering therapy with folic acid, vitamin B (12), and vitamin B (6) on clinical outcome after percutaneous coronary intervention: the Swiss Heart study: a randomized controlled trial. JAMA 2002;288 (8):973–79.

(43) Lange H, Suryapranata H, De Luca G, Borner C, Dille J, Kallmayer K, et al. Folate therapy and in-stent restenosis after coronary stenting. N Engl J Med 2004 Jun 24;350 (26):2673–81.

(44) Toole JF, Malinow MR, Chambless LE, Spence JD, Pettigrew LC, Howard VJ, et al. Lowering homocysteine in patients with ischemic stroke to prevent recurrent stroke, myocardial infarction, and death: the Vitamin Intervention for Stroke Prevention (VISP) randomized controlled trial. JAMA 2004 Feb 4;291 (5):565–75.

(45) Spence JD, Bang H, Chambless LE, Stampfer MJ. Vitamin Intervention for Stroke Prevention Trial: an efficacy analysis. Stroke 2005;36:2404–9.

(46) Salonen RM, Nyyssonen K, Kaikkonen J, Porkkala-Sarataho E,

Voutilainen S, Rissanen TH, et al. Six-year effect of combined vitamin C and E supplementation on atherosclerotic progression: the Antioxidant Supplementation in Atherosclerosis Prevention (ASAP) Study. Circulation 2003 Feb 25;107 (7):947–53.

(47) Lee IM, Cook NR, Gaziano JM, Gordon D, Ridker PM, Manson JE, et al. Vitamin E in the primary prevention of cardiovascular disease and cancer: the Women's Health Study: a randomized controlled trial. JAMA 2005 Jul 6;294 (1):56–65.

(48) Bailey DG, Spence JD, Munoz C, Arnold JM. Interaction of citrus juices with felodipine and nifedipine. Lancet 1991;337 (8736):268–69.

Index

Recipe listings and pages are typed in bold.